AN ATLAS OF ALIMENTARY TRACT PATHOLOGY

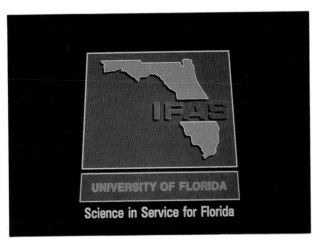
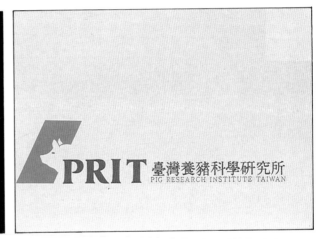

Claus D. Buergelt

Redman. M. Chu

Robert C.T. Lee

PIG RESEARCH INSTITUTE, TAIWAN
REPUBLIC OF CHINA
COLLEGE OF VETERINARY MEDICINE
UNIVERSITY OF FLORIDA U.S.A.

CONTENT

PREFACE

This atlas evolved from a series of lectures delivered to veterinary students at the University of Florida. It succeeds the two colored monographs on General Pathology edited by Drs. King and Lee and the Atlas of Cardiovascular Pathology edited by Drs. Liu, Hsu and Lee. All three volumes were published, printed and distributed by the Pig Research Institute, Taiwan and the Animal Industry Research Institute of Taiwan Sugar Corporation. The authors hope that this atlas will be part of a continuous series of colored monographs that focus on current and important diseases of special organ systems in domestic and other animal species.

The atlas is intended for veterinary pathologists, for practitioners who might need to interpret pathologic changes without the help of a pathologist while performing necropsies in the field, for residents and professional students. Its main purpose is to serve as a concise text-atlas for commonly encountered pathologic alterations in the alimentary tract. The emphasis is on the recognition of gross changes which are exemplified by photographic documentations. The photographic plates are accompanied by a short text, and a listing of references follows each chapter. The format largely follows the sequence in which individual organs of the alimentary tract are examined and described. Pathologic descriptions are used freely. The atlas is our perceptions of a rapidly expanding, dynamic and vast body of knowledge of alimentary track diseases.

The case collections have been from both, the University of Florida and the Pig Research Institute, Taiwan. Many people, in particular, Dr. John King, Cornell University, have directly and indirectly contributed to the contents of the atlas. We are much indebted to their contributions.

Our special thanks are extended to Iowa State University Press for agreeing to function as sole distributor of the atlas. It is hoped that the distributor's efforts will assist the authors in attractiong the greatest possible readership.

Claus D. Buergelt, DVM, PhD
Redman M. Chu, DVM, PhD
Robert C.T. Lee, DVM, PhD

ACKNOWLEDGEMENTS

This atlas is the product of combined illustrative and teaching resources from the contributing institutions: the Pig Research Institute, Taiwan and the University of Florida. Most of the material presented is complementary and provided from the collections of both facilities. However, the atlas would not have accomplished its objectives and reached completeness without the many valuable contributions from various friends, donors and associates. The one person helping with most of the added material was our friend and teacher John M. King, Cornell University. It is with utmost appreciation and gratitude that we would like to acknowledge and thank Dr. King for his selfless kodachrome contributions which were too numerous to list.

We would like to express our sincere gratitude and appreciation to the following individual and institutional contributors:

Dr. St. Barthold, Yale University   Plate 412

Dr. M. Chang, PRIT   Plate 263

Dr. Y.T. Chiu, PRIT   Plates 433,434,435,458

Dr. D. Forrester, University of Florida   Plate 164

Dr. R.O. Jacoby, Yale University   Plates 407,408

Dr. A. Lewis, Animal Medical Center   Plate 409

Dr. E. Momotani, Tsukula, Japan   Plate 201

Dr. H. Moon, NADC   Plate 192

Dr. J. Pohlenz, Hannover Veterinary College   Plates 192,194,195

Dr. L. Roth, Angel Memorial Hospital   P91,117,163,419

University of California   Plates 43,48,49,53,55,401,531

University of Missouri   Plates 8,15,16,33,118,135,281,287,289,303,307,343,366,367,368,
                        405,406,512

USDA FADD   Plate 23

The following plates were reproduced by permission of the journals listed below:

Journal of the American Veterinary Medical Association.

Volume 172:443-448,1978   Plates 196,197,264,272,322

The New England Journal of Medicine.

Volume 297:767-773,1977   Plates 199,200

Volume 325:327-340,1991   Plate 203

Scientific American, Volume 245:154-176,1981   Plates 191,193

The authors wish to gratefully acknowledge the assistance of the Taiwanese printing company and the valuable service offered by Iowa State University Press to function as marketing outlet for the atlas. Special thanks are extended to the Pig Research Institute, Taiwan for making the atlas possible and to the Council of Agriculture, Taiwan, and the College of Veterinary Medicine, University of Florida for support of the publication.

We are grateful to Mrs. Jennifer Maynard and Mrs. Marie Simmons, Miss Ing-Jen Sheu and Miss Daffodil Huang for assisting in the typing and to Drs. M. Chang and R.Z. Loung for assisting in the editing of the atlas.

Finally, special thanks to Mrs. Nancy Buergelt for encouragement and to our colleagues at PRIT for sharing their interest in our work.

INTRODUCTION

The specialty of gastroenterology has assembled a great body of knowledge during this past century. Die-tary corrections, the identification of attack mechanisms for various agents and toxins, the recognition of mechanistic categories involved in the pathogenesis of diarrhea and the mapping of the gut immune system as one of the largest defense systems in the body have made important contributions to the cause-and-effect relationships of primary gastroenteric diseases in both man and animals.

While many alimentary diseases are preventable due to available protective medications and vaccines and due to improved management or feeding practices, others keep occurring be it simply the result of anatomic and genetic species peculiarities that facilitate susceptibility to specific disease causes with very little chance towards prevention of occurrence at the present time. In frequency, diseases of the alimentary system are second to disorders of the skin. More importantly, great economic losses may be inflicted to the various animal industries from alimentary tract disorders that occur individually or as herd outbreaks on a larger scale. The necessity to quickly indentify the cause(s) of enteric diseases through trageted clinical examination and distinct morphological identification after death at the necropsy level is paramount to prevent spread and devastating losses.

The scope of this atlas is not intended to have the answers and solution to all gastrointestinal disease entities that presently occur in our domestic animal species. It logically is the next edition to the preceding volumes started by Drs. John M. King and Singkwan Liu at the National Pig Research Institute, Taiwan. As such, it is intended for a readership that is at the forefront to cope with gastrointestinal animal diseases, e.g. veterinary clinicians, veterinary pathologists, veterinary gastroenterologists and veterinary trainees. As reference it will be of use to meat inspectors, diagnostic laboratories, agriculture students, biologists, and libraries.

The atlas mainly contains illustrations of enteric diseases at the macroscopic level. Supplemental diagrams and cartoons should facilitate the recognition of major physiological and pathogenetic principles. The incorporation of schematic aspects of the enteric immune system is intended to illustrate different ways of the target tissue to react to the presence of infectious agents and antigens. The atlas is divided into five (5) chapters - diseases of the oral cavity; diseases of the esophagus; diseases of the forestomachs and stomachr; diseases of the small and large intestines; diseases of the peritoneum. Each chapter heading carries a brief introduction of the topic, followed by representative plates. The descriptive hallmarks are summarized for each plate. The sequence of the plates is similar for each of the five chapters and will concentrate on malformations, changes in position, primary degenerations, primary inflammations, endoparasites, neoplasms and miscellaneous disorders. The atlas mainly focuses on enteric diseases affecting domestic mammalian animal species. When appropriate. diseases affecting birds and laboratory animals are included. The atlas does not contain diseases of the liver and pancreas.

We do not claim completeness for our presentation of the topic. For detailed information we refer to recent textbooks and publications on alimentary tract animal diseases.

GLOSSARY

Achalasisa	Failure to relax
Brachygnathia	Abnormal growth of jaw bones
Braxy	Clostridial disease of sheep (ruminants)
Colic	Acute abdominal pain
Diarrhea	Abnormal frequency and liquidy of fecal discharge
Dysentery	Inflammation of intestine with abnormal pain, tenesmus and frequent stool containing blood and mucus
Dysphagia	Disorder of swallowing
Endotoxin	Heat-stable lipopolysaccharide with pyrogenic properties.
Enterocyte	Absorptive epithelium of intestine
Enterolith	Intestinal calculus
Eversion	Turning inside out of hollow organ
Exotoxin	Heat-labile protein with antigenic properties
Fetor ex ore	Halitosis
Hemomelasma Ilei	Blood-associated blackening of ileum
Lymphangiectasia	Dilatation of lymphatic vessels
Noma (Cancrum oris)	Gangrenous stomatitis caused by spirochetes and fusiform bacteria
Odontodystrophy	Dental anomalies
Phytobezoar	Concretion (ball) composed of fibers
Succus entericus	Liquid secreted by glands in the wall of the small intestine
Torsion	Twist of hollow organ upon its own longitudinal axis
Trichobezoar	Concretion (ball) composed of hair
Tympany	Abnormal collection of gas
Volvulus	Twist of hollow organ upon axis of its suspension (mesentery)

Chapter 1   The Oral Cavity

I.   Anomalies of Development

The development of a normal oral cavity depends on the integrated growth of a large number of embryologic processes.   Failures of integration and of fusion may lead to a variety of malformations; the most frequent ones are listed as follows.

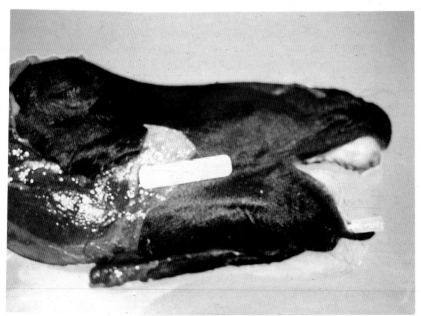

Plate 1   Brachygnathia.

Defined as an anomaly of the growth of the jaws.   Brachygnathia superior is the result of an abbreviation of the maxillae and is seen in brachycephalic dogs, in swine and cattle.   It is also known as "undershot".   Brachygnathia inferior is the result of an abbreviation of the mandibles and is commonly referred to as "overshot" or "parrot mouth".   A severe form of brachygnathia inferior has been reported in Shorthorn calves.   This is an "overshot" jaw in a premature foal.

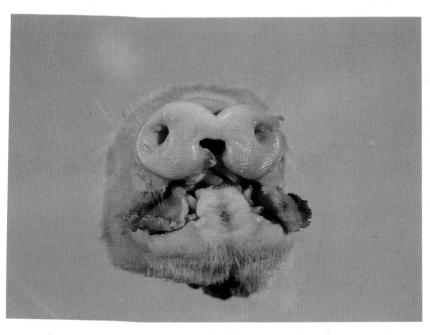

Plate 2   Facial Fissures and Clefts (Harelip)

A cleft lip may be unilateral or bilateral and may extend into the nostril or involve the maxillae.   This pig has a double tongue in addition.

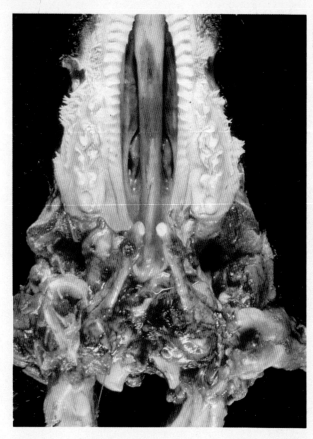

Plate 3   Cleft Palate (Palato-schisis)

Cleft palate results from inadequate growth of the palatine shelf and leaves a central defect that communicates with the oral and nasal cavities. Inability of affected animals to nurse properly and milk exuding from the nose at time of nursing are indicative of cleft palate; inhalation pneumonia is a common complication. Cleft palate may be associated with clefts of the lip and nostrils.

Plates 4,5   Cyclopia

Cyclops refers to the presence of a single, large median eye. Malformations of the oral cavity are additional complications. The condition is sporadically seen in pigs and calves. A wide range of cyclopia-type malformations occur endemically in lamb fetuses in the western states of the United States as the result of the consumption of the plant Veratrum californicum by pregnant ewes during early pregnancy. Prolonged gestation due to pituitary agenesis or hypoplasia is another complication factor in lambs carried by ewes grazing on Veratrum californicum. The cyclops in the piglet is a spontaneous malformation.

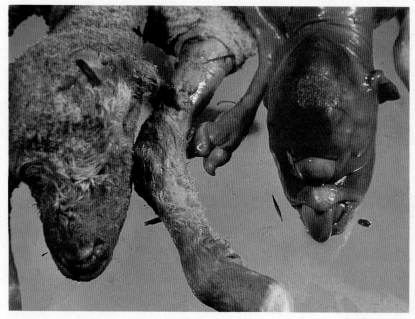

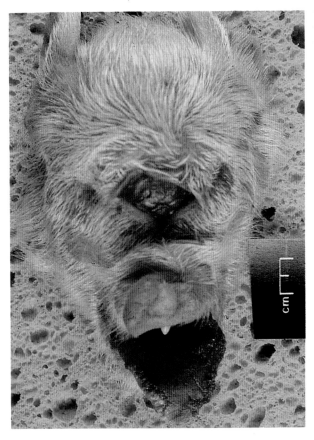

Plate 5   Cyclopia

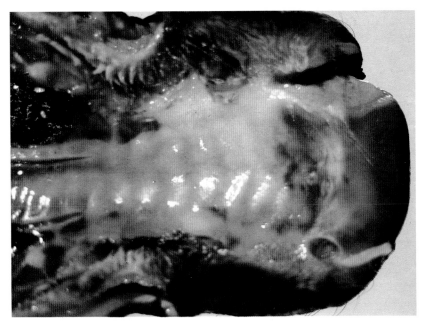

Plates 6,7   Epitheliogenesis Imperfecta

Several epithelial defects are present on the hard palate and tongue of this calf's mouth. As with the condition in the skin, these defects open up avenues towards secondary infection.

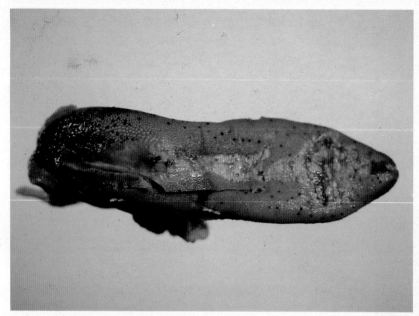

Plate 7   Epitheliogenesis Imperfecta

II.   Diseases of the Buccal Cavity and Tongue
Circulatory Disturbances

Certain systemic diseases associated with peripheral circulatory abnormalities become manifest within the mucous membranes of the oral cavity.   Observations such as pallor, cyanosis, petechiae, congestion and yellow discoloration are important clues with regard to the presence of specific disease entities. Careful examination of the oral mucosa is necessary for both clinicians and pathologists.

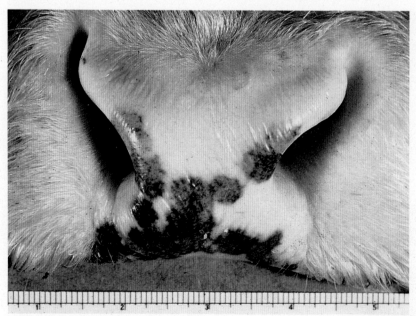

Plate 8   Pallor
White membranes and nares suggest blood loss or deficient bone marrow function.   This cow suffered from anemia resulting from abomasal haemonchosis.

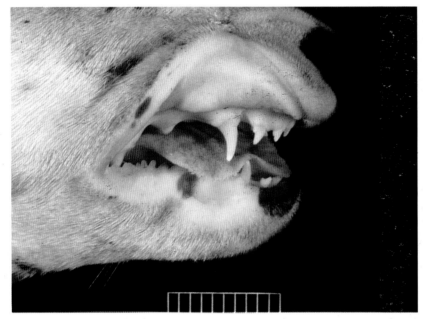

Plate 9 Icterus

This sheep died from copper toxicosis. Blood dyscrasias should be considered as differential diagnosis for yellow mucous membranes.

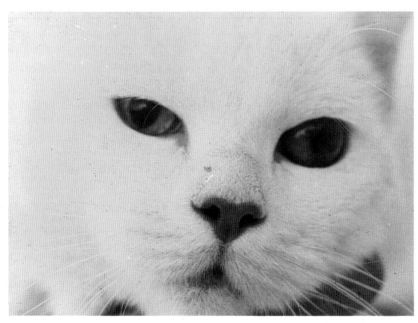

Plate 10 Cyanosis

Inadequate perfusion or insufficient oxygen supply are responsible for blue mucous membranes.

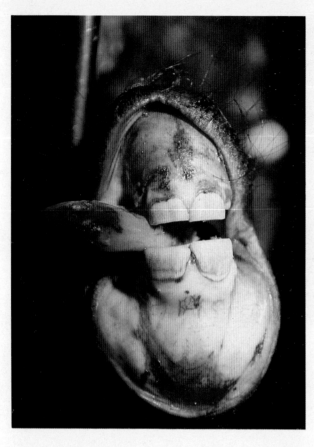

Plate 11   Petechiations
The changes support the diagnosis of septicemia, toxemia, thrombocytopenia, vascular permeability disturbances and treatment with non-steroidal antiinflammatory drugs as was the case in this foal.

Inflammations

Stomatitis denotes inflammation of the oral cavity. Glossitis denotes inflammation of the tongue, cheilitis that of the lips. Similar to color deviations of a normally pink oral mucosa, the recognition of certain types of inflammation may be extremely informative with regard to the presence of a specific disease. Based on the character of the exudate and the loss of integrity of the oral mucosa the following types of stomatitis are distinguished:

Catarrhal	Diphtheritic
Vesicular	Phlegmonous
Erosive	Purulent
Ulcerative	Papular

a.   Catarrhal

Catarrhal stomatitis is a superficial inflammation of the oral mucosa with evidence of edema, hyperemia and excessive mucus and saliva production. It is frequently the result of rough feed, heat, chemical burns and other irritants. Its healing tendency is excellent.

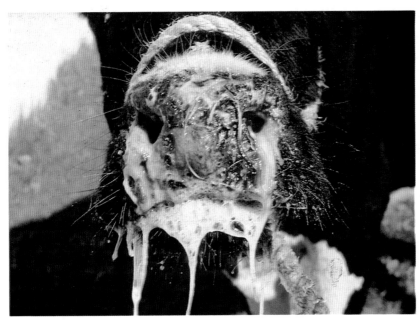

Plate 12 Excessive Salivation

Several causes should be considered differentially from local inflammations due to choke and systemic diseases such as rabies. This animal suffered from Malignant Catarrhal Fever.

b. Vesicular

The formation of vesicles filled with serous fluid denotes the prototype of a blistering stomatitis. Rupture of vesicles with transition to erosions occurs rapidly. Healing and regeneration are accomplished by an intact basal germinative layer. The identification of vesicular diseases may become very important in horses. cattle and swine as shall be seen from the following examples of virally induced stomatitides.

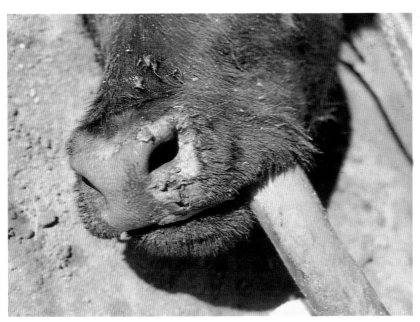

Plate 13 Foot and Mouth Disease (Aphthous Fever)

This economically important infection of ruminants and swine is caused by an aphthovirus. Seven major viral types are distinguished; the common ones are designated as A,O,C. The disease is characterized by an incubation period of 3 — 6 days and by clinical signs such as lameness and fever. There is an appreciable loss of weight and the oral cavity contains excessive saliva. Human infection is possible. Hyperemia. serous transudate, vesicles. bullae. erosions. mucopurulent exudate and scabs are visible pathological features within the oral cavity. Similar lesions occur in interdigital spaces around the coronets. teats, udder and the rumen. In pigs. the lesions are more common on the feet than in the oral cavity. They may be present, however, on the mouth and in the anterior nares.

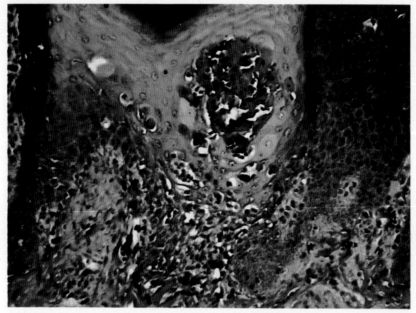

Plate 14 Foot and Mouth Disease

The histological target of the virus is the stratum spinosum. The cells of the stratum spinosum swell, develop eosinophilia of the cytoplasm and dissociate by vacuolar degeneration and retraction of the intercellular bridges. Interstitial fluid accumulates between the cell walls which are infiltrated by leukocytes. Later on, the cells of the outer stratified layers become hydropic and lyse. The early microvesicles coalesce to form macroscopically visible vesicles. These in turn may coalesce to form bullae. This microscopic description will serve as the prototype for all other virally induced vesicular disease to follow. GMS stain.

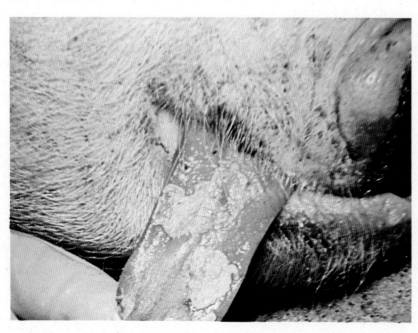

Plate 15 Vesicular Stomatitis (VS)

This specific viral disease occurs naturally in ruminants, swine and horses. It is caused by a vesiculovirus and is morphologically indistinguishable from foot and mouth disease. It mainly affects the oral cavity and is of economic importance where it regularly occurs. Its occurrence in North America is sporadic. In cattle, foot lesions are less common, but this is by no means a dependable feature. Outbreaks of the disease in cattle have been described in which lesions were predominantly on the teats. The disease takes on a severe form in pigs.

Vesicular Exanthema (VE)

This viral disease occurs naturally only in swine. The virus has been also isolated from harbor seals in California. It is a member of the family Caliciviridae. Vesicles develop on the snout, lips, tongue, gingiva, and on the sole, coronary band and interdigital skin in swine.

Swine Vesicular Disease (SVD)

This picornavirus has been reported to cause stomatitis in the swine population of Europe and Hong Kong. Clinically, it cannot be distinguished from the above mentioned vesicular diseases. However, the disease has a central nervous component, such as non-purulent meningoencephalitis. Mice and men are susceptible to the virus as well.

c. Erosive-ulcerative

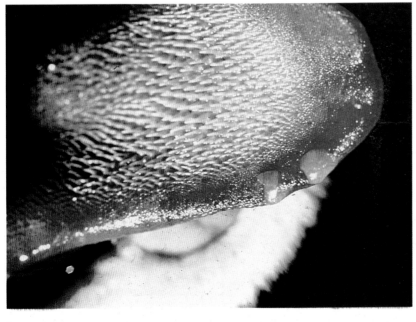

Plate 16   Feline Calicivirus Infection (FCV)

The virus is mainly responsible for acute respiratory infections in cats. Ocular involvement and ulcers on the tongue and hard palate accompany the respiratory lesions. The virus has been implicated to cause chronic stomatitis,though no increased isolation rate is found in affected cats when compared to uninfected cats. The evidence of the feline immunodeficiency virus (FIV) as co-agent is unclear.

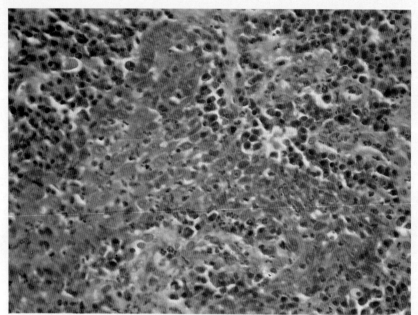

Plate 17   Chronic Feline Plasmacytic-Lymphocytic Gingivitis

Infection by specific bacteria or viruses is unlikely to be the cause. It is most likely a multifactorial disease in cats and resembles noma. A hypersensitivity reaction to an exogenous antigen(s) cannot be ruled out. The role of FCV, FIV and FeLV viruses as causative agents remains unclear. H&E stain.

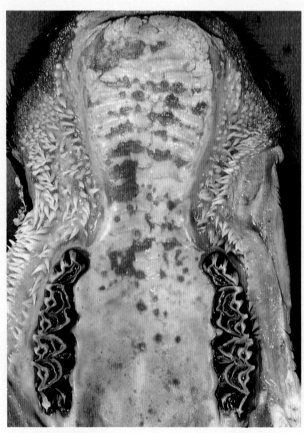

Plate 18   Bovine Virus Diarrhea (BVD)

Note erosions and hemorrhages of the oral mucosa of the hard palate. The pestivirus causes erosions,ulcerations and hemorrhages throughout the alimentary canal. Interdigital dermatitis, mummification, abortion and cerebellar hypoplasia of calves are additional pathological findings.Young animals between 6-14 months of age are usually affected. This disease has a febrile onset and causes watery diarrhea clinically.Characteristic pathological changes include:

Necrosis of the surface epithelium in upper alimentary tract (superficial layers); damage of crypt epithelium in small intestines; lymphatic necrosis of Peyer's patches; hyaline necrosis of small arteries of intestinal submucosa.

Infectious Bovine Rhinotracheitis, Malignant Catarrhal Fever or Bluetongue infection should be contenders for the differential diagnosis.

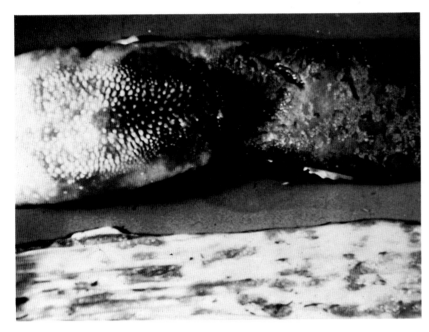

Plate 19   BVD

Sharp, punched-out linear erosions with hemorrhage in the esophagus are characteristically associated with BVD. The surface of the tongue is covered by a fibrinonecrotic exudate.

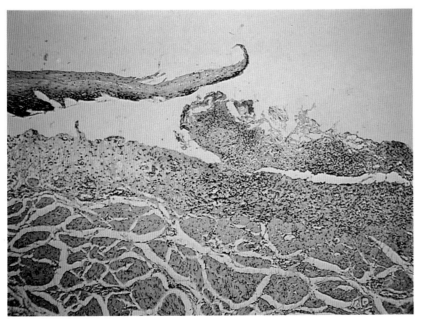

Plate 20   Esophagus with BVD

Histologically, the squamous epithelium is lifted off and demonstrates necrosis with inflammatory cells demarcating the exposed lamina propria. H&E stain.

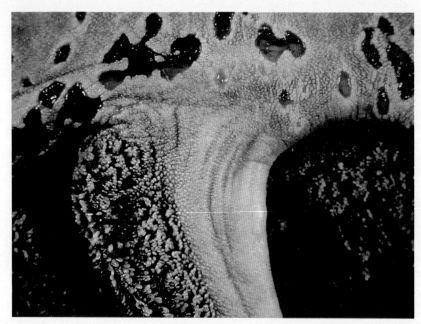

Plate 21
Ulcers with sharp margins are present on the pillars of the rumen.

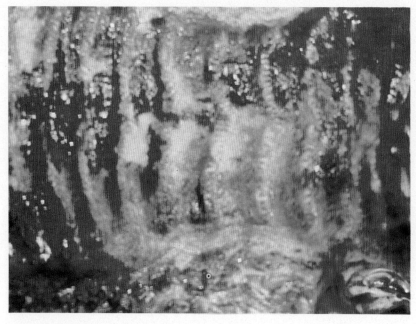

Plate 22 Bovine Malignant Catarrhal Fever (BMCF)
The disease is caused by a herpesvirus. Sheep and Wildebeest are natural agent reservoirs. Clinical signs are accompanied by fever and lymphadenopathy. There is nasal discharge, conjunctivitis and corneal edema. The disease occurs in four forms: nervous, ocular, intestinal and dermal. The forms may overlap. Catarrhal, mucopurulent, pseudomembranous and necrotic changes are observed along the various mucous membranes.

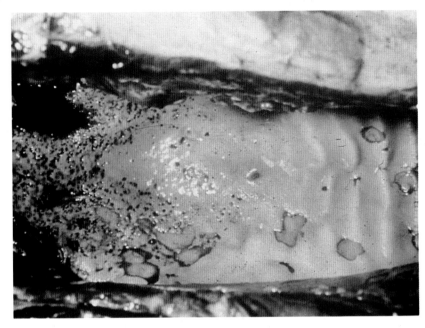

Plate 23　BMCF

Ulcerations of the tongue in BMCF.

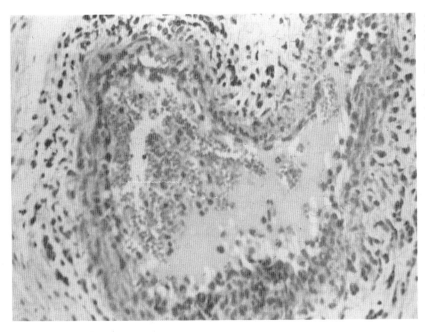

Plate 24　BMCF

Histologically, vasculitis with fibrinoid necrosis is pathognomonic for the diagnosis of BMCF at the morphologic level. H&E stain.

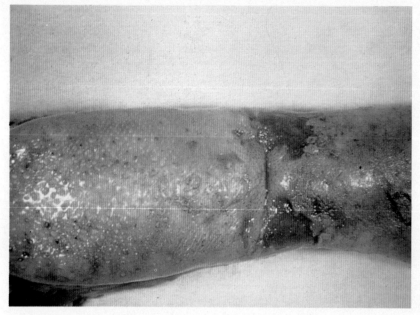

Plate 25 Bluetongue

This orbivirus affects ruminants, is transmitted by insects (Culicoides sp.)and has a strong vascular endothelial tropism. Hyperemia, edema, cyanosis,swelling of surface epithelium, petechiations, erosions and ulcerations are common findings. Mouth, lips, tongue, face, ears, nares, skin and feet(coronet perioplic band) are affected. The cyanotic appearance of the glossal mucosa is responsible for the name of the disease. The cause of the disease in cattle is milder than in sheep. Central nervous system lesions are observed in ovine fetuses. Subintimal hemorrhages of the aorta and pulmonary arteries support the diagnosis of bluetongue in sheep. Differential diagnoses should consider photosensitization, contagious ecthyma and sheep pox.

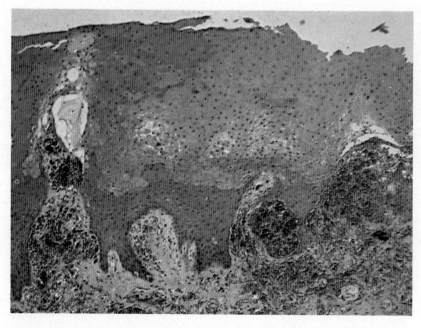

Plate 26 Bluetongue

Extravasation of red blood cells beneath the glossal papillae indicates vascular permeability disturbance.H&E stain

d. Papular

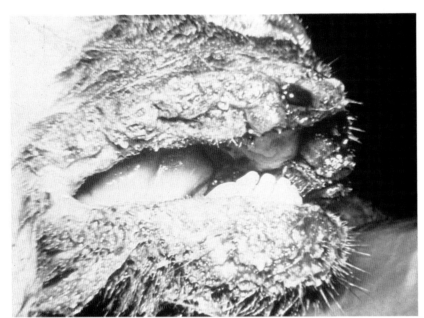

Plates 27,28   Contagious Ovine Ecthyma   (ORF)

This contagious parapoxvirus causes characteristic nodular lesions on lips, oral mucous membranes, udder and feet of sheep and goats. The disease must be differentiated from sheep pox and ulcerative dermatosis. The virus is transmissible to humans.

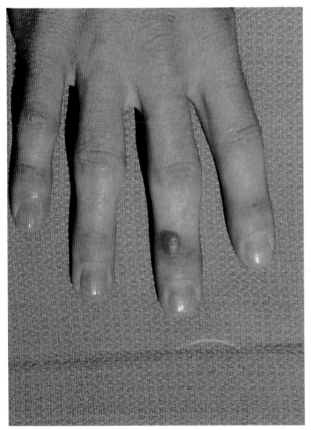

Plate 28   Contagious Ovine Ecthyma

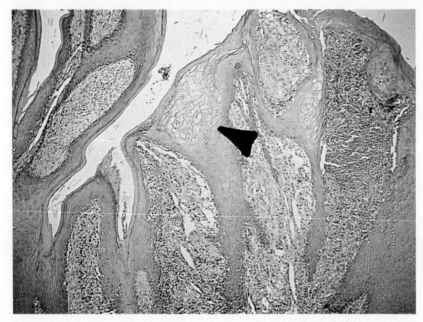

Plate 29   Contagious Ovine Ecthyma

Observe proliferative epithelium with rete pegs. ballooning degeneration (arrow) and inflammatory exudate in submucosa in sheep suffering from "scabby mouth" H&E stain.

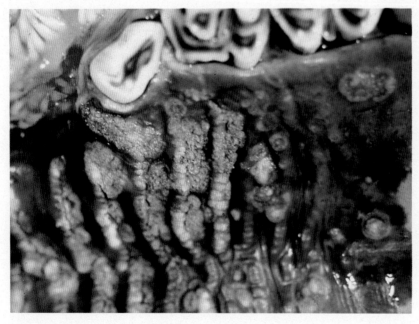

Plate 30   Bovine Papular Stomatitis

A mild viral disease with raised lesions in and around the mouth and muzzles of young cattle occurs sporadically in Europe and in North America and may simulate some features of other important infectious bovine diseases. The parapoxvirus is closely related to paravaccinia (pseudo-cowpox virus) and also to ORF. It is transmissible to man. The papular lesions may ulcerate and ultimately heal.

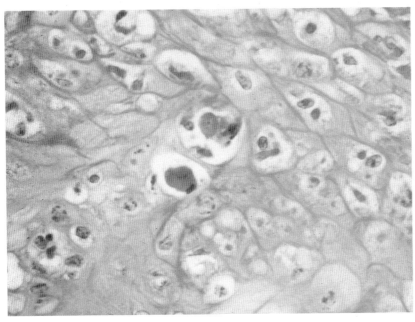

Plate 31 Bovine Papular Stomatitis

Histologically, the stratum spongiosum is spongiotic and contains cytoplasmic inclusions. Epithelial nuclei may undergo pyknosis. H&E stain.

e. Diphtheritic

The formation of pseudomembranes as the result of fibrinous exudation and necrosis of surface structures and an underlying inflammatory response characterize this type of stomatitis. The lesions may be quite extensive and may involve deep tissues of the oral cavity. Calves, lambs and young pigs are primarily affected. Opportunistic pyogenic bacteria such as Fusobacterium necrophorum, Actinomyces pyogenes and Spirochetes are commonly isolated. Predisposing trauma and other infectious diseases may set an invasive stage for the organisms. Diphtheritic inflammations frequently develop into excessive purulent inflammations. Abscesses and chronic fistulae may follow.

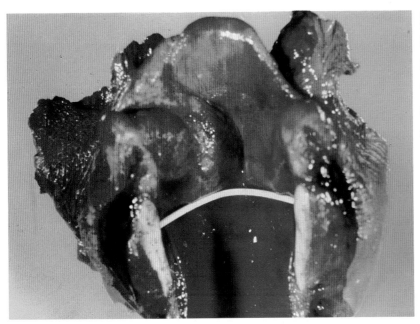

Plate 32 Oral Necrobacillosis

Fibrinonecrotic glossitis, pharyngitis and laryngitis may develop in calves infected with F. necrophorum. The disease is also known as "calf diphtheria". Death may occur acutely from septicemia.

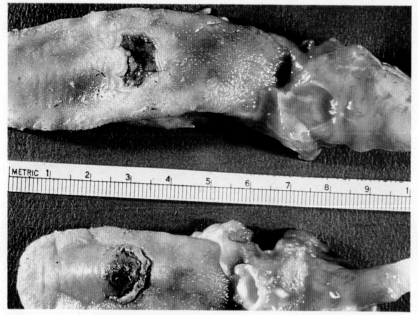

Plate 33   Glossal Necrobacillo-sis
Self-inflicted trauma from wrongly clipped teeth caused secondary infection with F. necrophorum in these piglets.

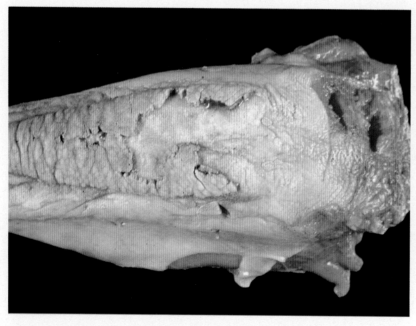

Plate 34   Candidiasis
The slide illustrates candidiasis (thrush) affecting the dorsal surface of the tongue of a foal.Candidiasis occurs most common-ly in young animals.debilitated patients and as a complication of protracted an-tibiotic therapy. The gross lesions are characterized by a crusty, tan pseudomem-branes overlying the mucous membranes.

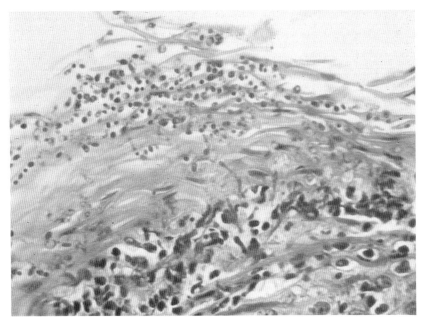

Plate 35   Candidiasis

Microscopically, the pseudomembrane is composed of masses of fibrin and of pseudohyphae of invading Candida yeasts. H&E stain.

f.   Phlegmonous – granulomatous

These forms are examples of deep stomatitides.

Plate 36   Actinobacillosis

Actinobacillus lignieresii, a gram-negative bacillus normally inhabits the skin and oral cavity of cattle. It is the etiologic agent which, after abrasions of the mucous membranes, causes a granulomatous tissue response. The distribution is best seen beneath the mucosa of the dorsal and the lateral surfaces of the tongue.

As the granulomatous response is associated with sclerosing processes the disease is referred to as "wooden tongue". Although actinobacillosis in cattle is best known as a disease of the tongue, the infection may occur in any of the exposed soft tissues of the mouth and neck. The infection is of low spread, but clinically may result in dysphagia, excessive salivation, pharyngeal stenosis and respiratory distress.

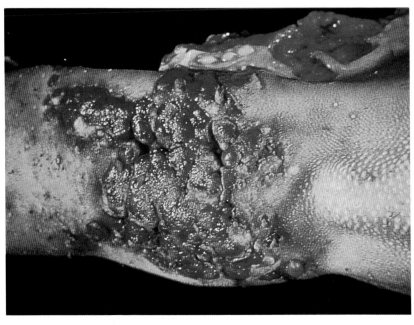

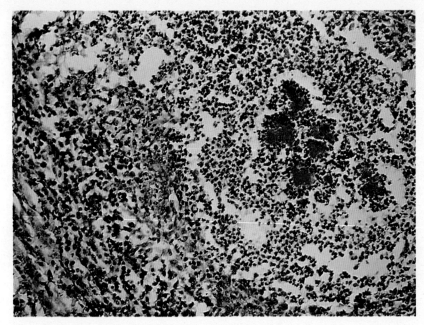

Plate 37 Actinobacillosis

Microscopically, actinobacillosis is characterized by a pyogranulomatous inflammation containing discrete colonies of organisms surrounded by radiating clubs suspended in neutrophils and encapsulated by dense connective tissue. Goodpasture stain.

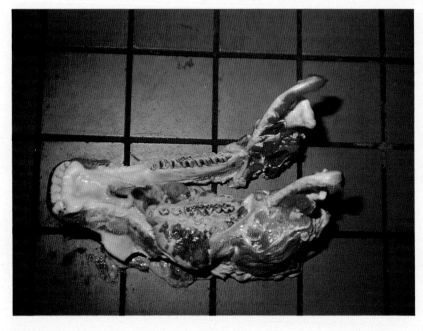

Plate 38 Actinomycosis

Actinomycosis, a disease of similar pathogenesis, is caused by a gram-positive, anaerobic organism, Actinomyces bovis. The bacillus invades oral soft tissues and the underlying jaw,usually the mandibles.

III. Diseases of the Teeth.

Dental diseases in animals are frequently overlooked. They may be contributory to or the single cause of cachexia.

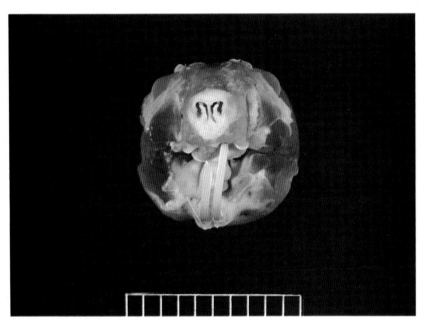

Plate 39   Irregularities in Wear

Dental malocclusion is a common problem in caged laboratory animals as depicted in this rat. Abnormalities of wearing are also common in herbivores. Excessive wear may be encountered in horses. Abnormal wear can be due to abnormal chewing as the result of painful foreign bodies or fractures.

Pigmentations

The dentin may be discolored yellowish in icterus; pink in cats, cows or pigs as the result of congenital porphyria; brownish after chronic fluorosis or black adjacent to the gums as the result of deposition of lead sulfur in chronic lead poisoning (lead seam).

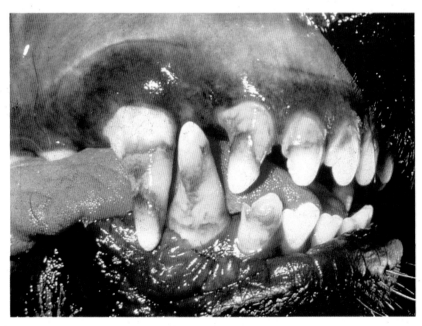

Plate 40   Odontodystrophy in Canine Distemper

Hypoplasia or loss of the enamel is caused by a variety of systemic disturbances such as malnutrition, fluorine poisoning, vitamin A deficiencies or infectious disease, for example canine distemper.

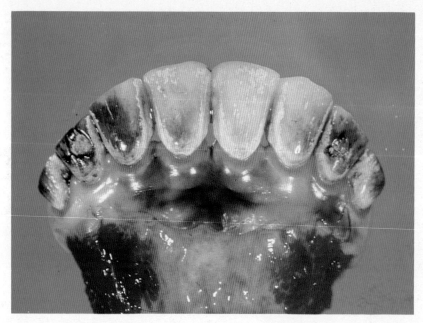

Plate 41 Chronic Fluorosis

Excessive greenish-black, yellow or brown mottling of bovine teeth is characteristic of chronic fluorosis. Other changes in the teeth include chalky, excessive attrition and hypoplastic pitting of the enamel. Chronic poisoning of this nature occurs in animals eating pasturage or range contaminated by airborne residues from aluminum manufacturers, phosphate refineries and similar industrial installations, or drinking well water containing soluble fluorides in significant quantity. Fluor is resorbed from the rumen and incorporated into bones and teeth. Developing teeth reveal enamel discoloration or defects and foster wear and tear.

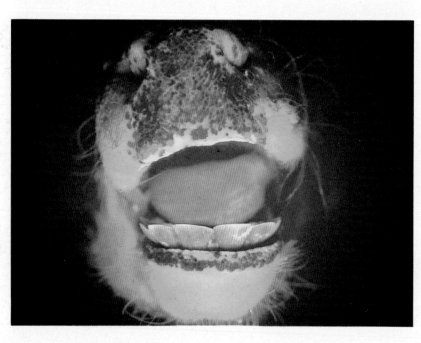

Plate 42 Congenital Porphyria

"Pink tooth" in a cow with congenital porphyria which is a metabolic defect affecting the synthesis of the normal heme pigment, ferroprotoporphyrin,resulting in the release of abnormal amounts of free porphyrins into serum and tissues. The accumulation of porphyrins leads to photosensitization when cattle are exposed to strong fluorescence. Genetic data indicate that porphyria is inherited as an autosomal recessive trait in cattle and as an autosomal dominant trait in cats and swine.

Dental Calculus (Tartar) and Caries

These are major dental diseases in man. They are also common findings in older dogs and cats and may lead to "fetor ex ore". Tartar is a composite calcified mass of bacteria, fungi, food particles, desquamated epithelium and inflammatory cells. Caries is the result of destructive decalcification of dentin followed by enzymatic lysis of exposed organic matrix. It is due to organic acids (lactic acid) which are produced by peptonizing bacteria.

Dental Inflammations

Pulpitis refers to inflammation of the soft connective tissue core of the tooth. It is associated with bacterial infection which may spread to surrounding bones. Periodontitis is inflammation of the surrounding soft tissues. It may be superficial and is then referred to as gingivitis or it may involve deeper structures and is then referred to as pyorrhea. Continued irritation may cause hyperplasia, metaplasia and occasionally neoplasia (squamous cell carcinoma) of gingival mucosal epithelium.

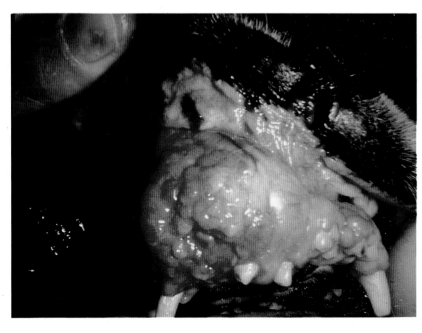

Plates 43,44 Gingival Hyperplasia – Epulis Complex

The term "epulis" describes a localized tumorous enlargement of gingival tissue closely associated with the periodontal ligament. This mass can be composed of both a true benign tumor and of exuberant stromal tissue derived from chronic irritation. The specific neoplastic part has also been called fibromatous epulis or osseous epulis of periodontal origin because of the bone, cementum or dentin that it generally contains. These growths are common in dogs of all ages and are frequently located in the premolar and molar regions. Though considered morphologically benign, local recurrence following excision is frequently seen. The overlying gingival mucosa is markedly thickened due to rete pegs. H&E stain.

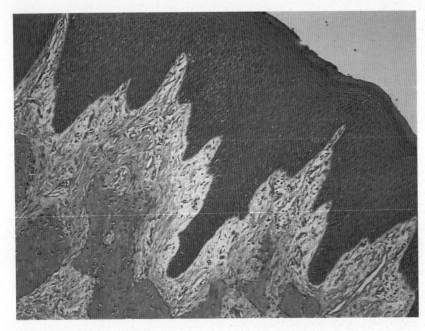

**Plate 44   Gingival Hyperplasia –
Epulis Complex**

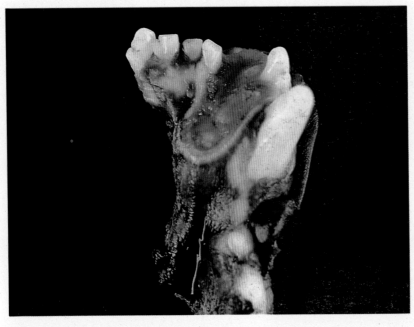

Plate 45   Acanthomatous Epulis

Unlike fibromatous epulis or osseous epulis, acanthomatous epulis of periodontal ligament origin infiltrates and destroys the periodontal apparatus, including the alveolar bone. Acanthomatous epulis is sensitive to radiation therapy. It may recur following excision.

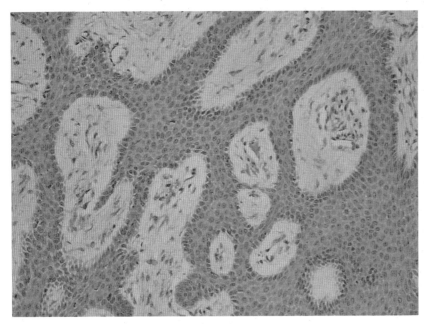

Plate 46 Acanthomatous Epulis

Sheets of epithelial cells are palisading, interdigitating and spreading within fibrous matrix. Lack of keratinization differentiates it from squamous cell carcinoma.H&E stain

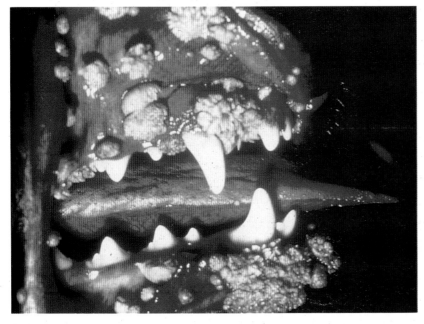

Plate 47 Canine Oral Papillomatosis

Oral papillomas in young dogs are caused by a virus and are considered contagious. Unlike dermal papillomas, the disease is followed by spontaneous regression. Intranuclear and cytoplasmic inclusions can be present.

IV. Neoplasms of the Oral Cavity

A variety of neoplastic infiltrations occur in dogs and cats, and occasionally in horses. The proper morphologic identification and classification of the neoplasms is important for various therapeutic interventions. Proliferative inflammatory processes and the gingival hyperplasia-epulis complex have to be considered as differential diagnoses. Sites of importance in the dog, in order of frequency, are gingiva, tonsil, lip, cheek and palate, whereas in the cat, they are the gingiva and tongue. In dogs, carcinomas and melanomas are the most common neoplasms, while fibrosarcomas are less frequent. In cats, carcinomas are the most common neoplasms. Benign oral-pharyngeal neoplasms exclusive infectious papilloma and periodontal epulis are rare.

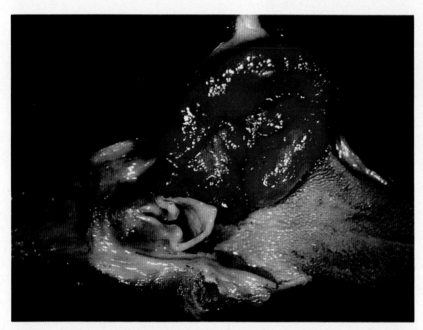

Plate 48 Squamous Cell Carcinoma of Tonsil

Tonsillar squamous cell carcinomas are more frequent in dogs, whereas those of the tongue occur more commonly in cats. Squamous cell carcinomas of the tonsils have a high propensity to metastasize, and the prognosis is poor.

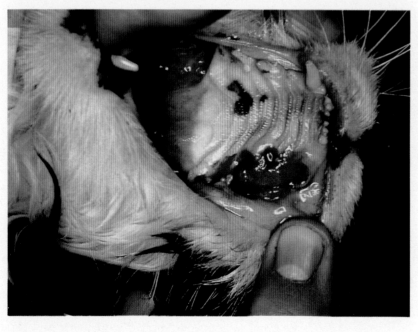

Plate 49 Squamous Cell Carcinoma of Gingiva

The neoplasm invades locally destroying palatine and periodontal structures including bone.

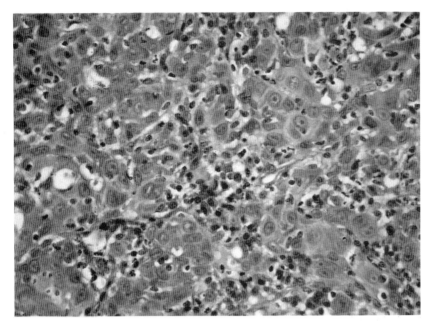

Plate 50　Squamous Cell Carcinoma

Cords of neoplastic squamous cell invade the underlying soft tissue. Keratin pearls and mitotic figures as well as interdigitations are common.H&E stain

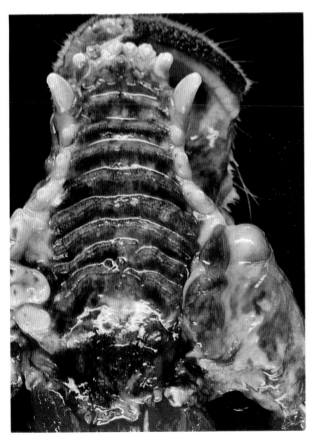

Plate 51　Oral Melanoma

The tumors become rapidly growing, firm black masses with a dome-shaped, smooth surface. Depending on the amount of melanin pigment present, the interior may be white, grey, dark brown or black. The vast majority of oral melanomas are malignant with metastases via lymphatics or blood vessels. The prognosis is very poor.

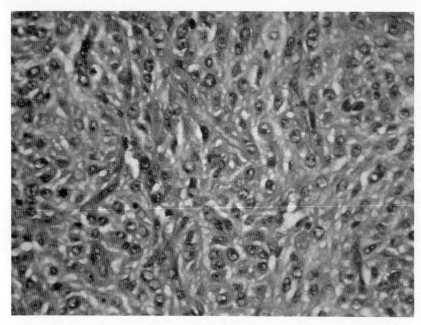

Plate 52   Oral Melanoma

Histologically. the tumor is composed of melanocytes carrying varying degrees of melanin in the cytoplasm. Epithelioid or spindle-cell types are recognized. The tumor cell may be amelanotic as in this case. but most amelanotic melanomas have a few clusters of pigmented cells. H&E stain.

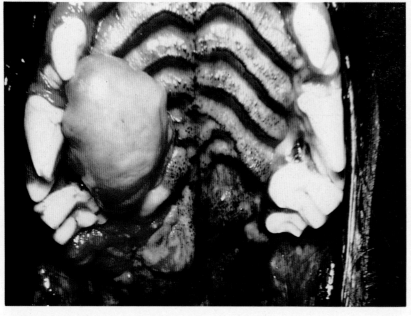

Plate 53   Oral Fibrosarcoma

The gum is the most common site for fibrosarcomas to occur in dogs. The tumors are solitary. firm with a smooth nodular surface. Despite the local invasion of bone. metastases are rare. The neoplasm has to be differentiated from epulis and oral lymphosarcomas.

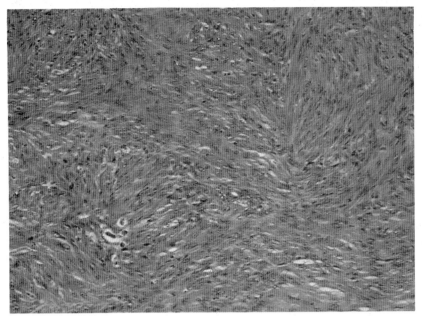

Plate 54 Oral Fibrosarcoma

Interwoven bundles of malignant spindle cells determine the diagnosis. H&E stain

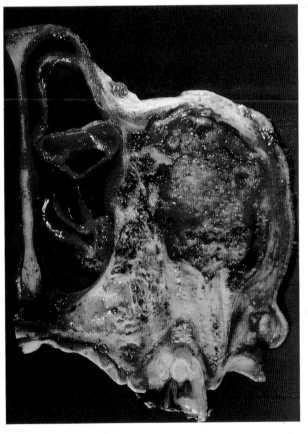

Plate 55 Ameloblastic Adamantinoma

This is a neoplasm of enamel origin invading the maxillary and nasal passages of a 4 year old horse. Most tumors of dental origin grow in an expansile fashion, tend to destroy bone and are difficult to remove.

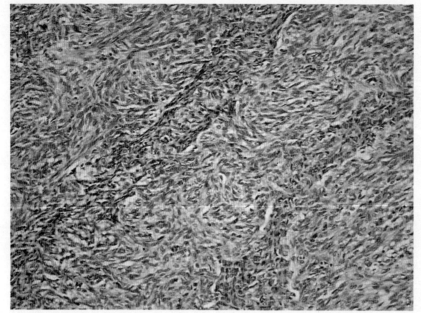

Plate 56　Ameloblastic Adamantinoma

Palisading ameloblastic epithelium is embedded in well-differentiated stellate reticulum.　Interbranching ribbons of elongated epithelial cells are present. The tumor needs to be differentiated from acanthomatous epulis and squamous cell carcinoma histologically. H&E stain

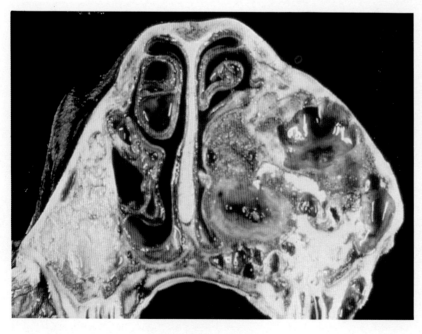

Plate 57　Odontoma

Odontomas are dental tumors in which all dental tissues are represented(enamel, dentin, cementum, pulp) and are always tumors of young dogs and horses.　This neoplasm in a young horse unilaterally occupies the nasal passages.

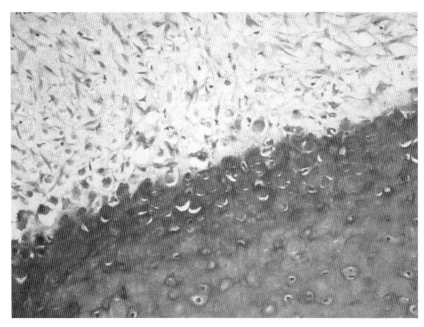

Plate 58 Odontoma

Microscopically, the neoplasm is composed of ameloblasts, odontoblasts and dental substance resembling cementum. H&E stain.

V. Miscellaneous

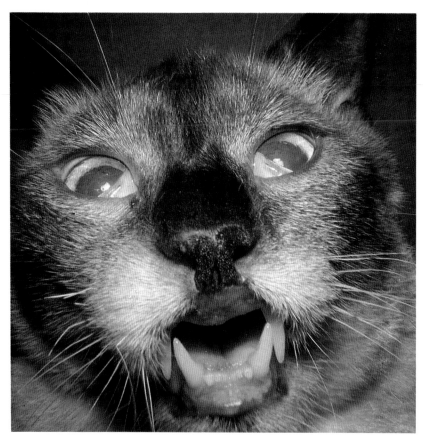

Plate 59   Eosinophilic Granuloma-Complex

This peculiar disease principally affects the upper and lower lips, the tongue, the oral mucosa and integument of cats and rarely of dogs. It is also known as "rodent ulcer" and may be spread to various dermal parts of the body by licking. Its etiology remains undetermined, but food allergy has been postulated as cause. Squamous cell carcinoma should be considered as differential diagnosis. Oral eosinophilic granulomas have been reported in Siberian Husky dogs.

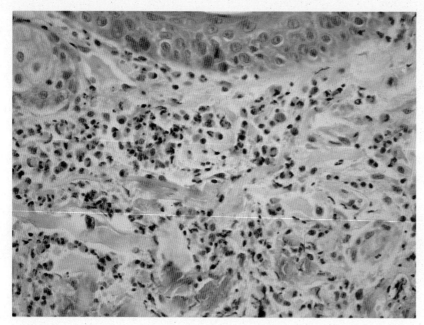

Plate 60 Eosinophilic Granuloma-Complex

The disease is histologically characterized by the presence of eosinophils, mast cells and macrophages. Focal collagenolysis may occur. H&E stain.

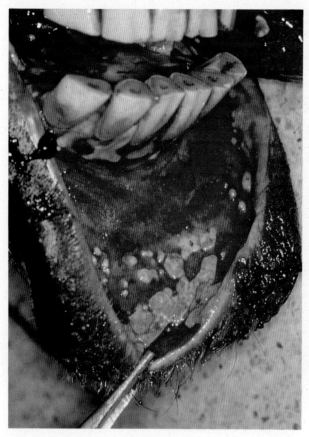

Plates 61-64 Pemphigus

Pemphigus is one type of immune-mediated blistering or bullous skin diseases of dogs, cats and horses that may extend to mucocutaneous junctions. It is currently thought that pemphigus develops by deposition of antibodies and complement components into intercellular spaces of the epidermis causing acantholysis. Bullae, erosions and ulcerations are gross features of this disease. Severe erosions are present in the oral mucous membranes and tongue of a horse with pemphigus vulgaris.

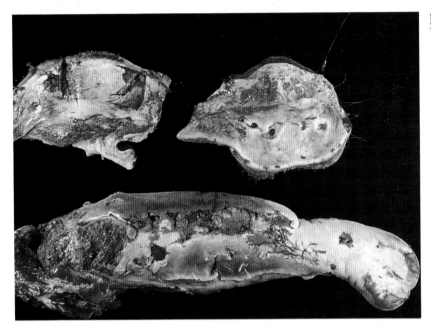

Plate 62   Pemphigus

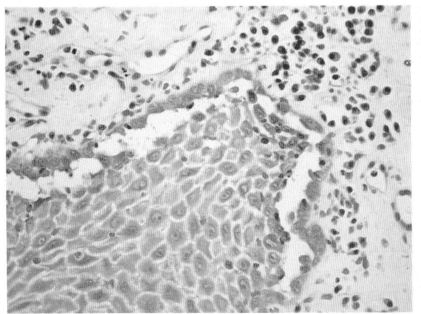

Plate 63   Pemphigus

Biopsy specimen from oral lesion of dog with pemphigus vulgaris demonstrating acantholysis of prickle cell layers of the oral mucosa.   Desmosomes have disappeared.   Suprabasilar clefts and "tombstone" appearance of the basal cells are additional features. H&E stain.

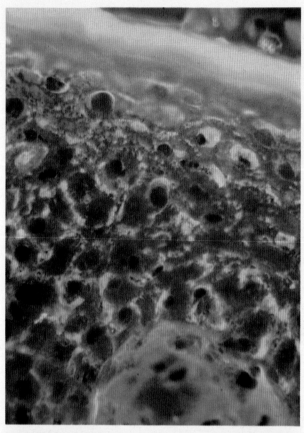

Plate 64　Pemphigus

Immunofluorescent staining is helpful to confirm the diagnosis. In a positive case, the intercellular cement substance of stratified squamous epithelium stains for serum antibodies and/or complement components in a linear pattern as demonstrated in this photomicrograph.

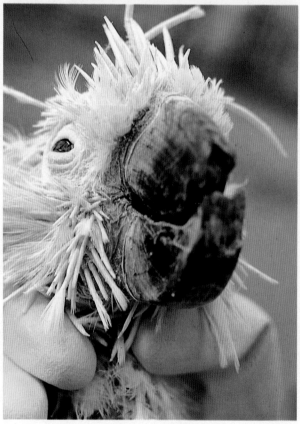

Plate 65　Psittacine Beak and Feather Disease (PBFD)

PBFD has been reported in numerous species of captive and wild psittacines. Clinical signs include depression, some diarrhea and widespread loss of feathers. Beak deformities are additional findings as depicted in a Moluccan Cockatoo.

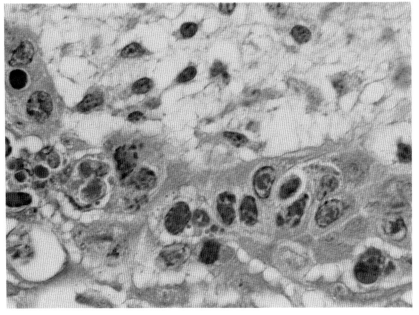

Plates 66,67   Psittacine Beak and Feather Disease

Microscopically, hemorrhage, necrosis, lymphocyte and heterophil infiltrations are present within the feather pulp cavity. Feather epithelial cells reveal focal necrosis and several have basophilic intranuclear inclusion bodies. Macrophages in the pulp cavity contain globular intracytoplasmic inclusion bodies. Electronmicrographs reveal these inclusions to contain parvovirus-like particles. H&E stain.

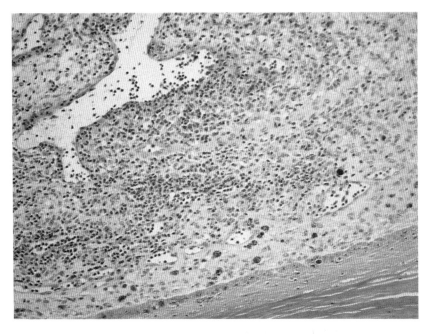

Plate 67   Psittacine Beak and Feather Disease

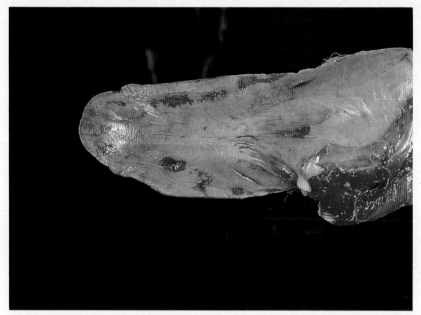

Plate 68 Uremic Glossitis

Focal necrosis, hemorrhage and ulcers on this dog's ventral tongue are associated with severe chronic uremia. The margins of the ulcer are swollen and they may become indurated. Halitosis is a good indicator for chronic renal disease.

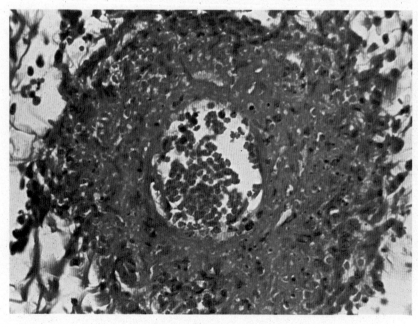

Plate 69 Uremic Glossitis

Fibrinoid necrosis and vasculitis are associated microscopic changes in chronic uremia. H&E stain.

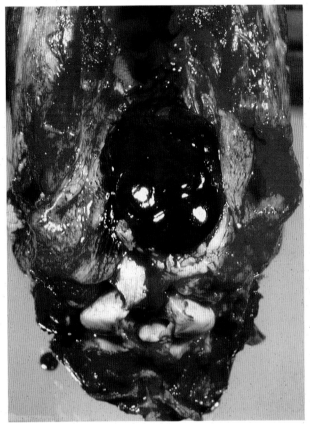

Plate 70   Guttural Pouch Mycosis

Sudden, massive epistaxis and hemoptysis in horses can be the result of erosive actions of mainly Aspergillus sp. invasion. Unilateral mycotic infection is the sequela to a preceding insult to the stylohyoid apparatus (luxation, fracture) and the anatomical proximity of the internal carotid artery, cranial nerves and the middle ear. Opportunistic fungi erode and thrombose the internal carotid artery leading to serious bleeding consequences.

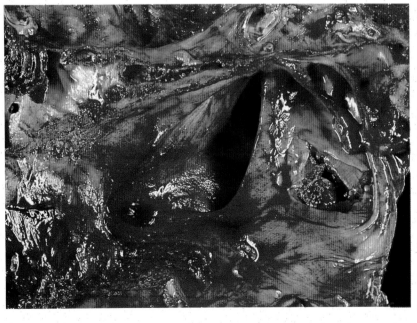

Plate 71   Guttural Pouch Empyema

Purulent exudate in the guttural pouch can result from concretions, strangles (Streptococcus equi) or Pythiosis. The genus Pythium, a member of the Oomycetes, belongs to the kingdom of Protista, and is now excluded from the true fungi. The causative organism has been established to be Pythium insidiosum, a new species. It is a plant parasite that inhabits wet environments and water-logged soils in tropical and subtropical climates. This would explain the occurrence of equine pythiosis on swampy land. In addition, human and canine cases have been reported. The disease in horses is characterized by rapidly enlarging, fistulating and ulcerating granulomas principally on the limbs, but sometimes on the head, ventral abdomen and genitalia. This particular equine case reveals pythiosis affecting the guttural pouch.

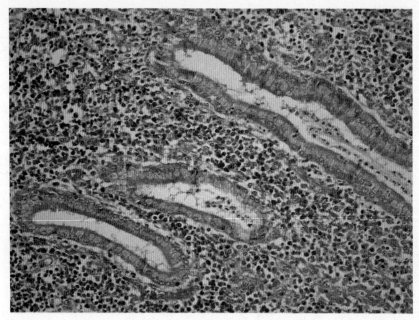

Plate 72 Guttural Pouch Pythio-sis

The microscopic presence of eosinophils and lymphocytes suggest presence of fungi. H&E stain.

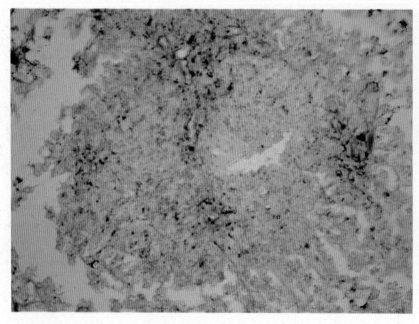

Plate 73 Guttural Pouch Pythio-sis

Broad, branching, aseptate hyphae within coagulation necrosis of soft tissue brings to light Pythium as causative organism. GMS stain.

Literature

1 . R.R. Dubielzig, and D.E. Thrall: Ameloblastoma and Keratinizing Ameloblastoma in Dogs. Vet. Path. 19: 596, 1982.

2 . S.J. Duffell, J.W. Hakness: Bovine Virus Diarrhea - Mucosal Disease Infection in Cattle. Vet. Res. 117: 240, 1985.

3 . C.E. Harvey: Oral Inflammatory Diseases in Cats. J. Am. An. Hosp. Assoc. 27:585, 1991.

4 . S.S. Lai, P.D. McKerchev, D.M. Moore, J.H. Gillespie: Pathogenesis of Swine Vesicular Disease in Pigs. Am. J. Vet. Res. 40:463, 1979.

5 . K.S. Latimer, P.M. Rakich, W.L. Steffens, I.M. Kircher, et al.: A Novel DNA Virus Associated with Feather Inclusions in Psittacine Beak and Feather Disease. Vet. Path. 28:300, 1991.

6 . H.D. Liggitt, J.C. DeMartini, A.E. McChesney et al.: Experimental Transmission of Malignant Catarrhal Fever in Cattle: Gross and Histopathologic Changes. Am. J. Vet. Res. 39:1249, 1978.

7 . K.E. Stebbins, C.C. Morse, M.H. Goldschmidt: Feline Oral Neoplasia: A 10-year Survey. Vet. Path. 26: 121, 1989.

8 . J.L. Shupe, R.H. Bruner, J.L. Seymour, C.L. Alden: The Pathology of Chronic Bovine Fluorosis. A Review. Toxicologic Pathol. 20:274, 1992.

9 . C. von Tscharner, B. Bigler: The Eosinophilic Granuloma Complex. J. Sm. An.Prac. 30:228, 1989.

Chapter 2   The Esophagus

As tubular organ, the esophagus provides the route of passage for masticated food to reach the stomach. It is divided into three anatomical parts: cervical, thoracic and abdominal. There are three anatomical narrowings: at the larynx, the thoracic inlet and the diaphragmatic hiatus. Esophageal diseases are relatively rare as compared to other compartments of the alimentary tract.

I.   Obstruction

Foreign objects or impactions may occlude the lumen of the esophagus. If the obstruction is not relieved soon, pressure necrosis and local gangrene develop. Predisposing factors are dental diseases, poor-quality feed and the presence of neuromotoric esophageal or gastric diseases.

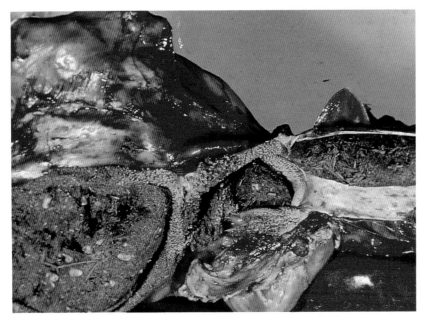

Plate 74   Impaction

Food impaction in the lower portion of the esophagus in a sheep as the result of ruminal impaction.

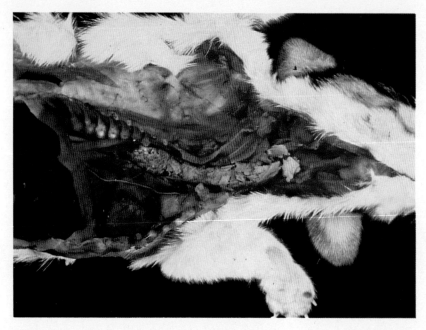

Plate 75 Impaction

Wood shavings impaction of the esophagus in a puppy.

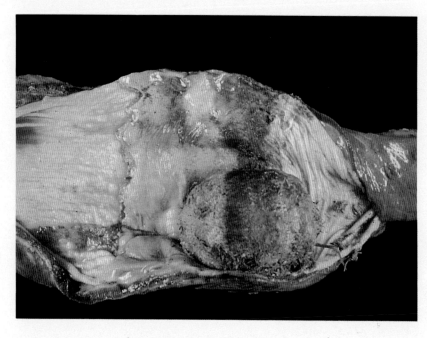

Plate 76 Choke

Necrosis of the esophageal mucosa at point of foreign body obstruction (choke) in a horse.

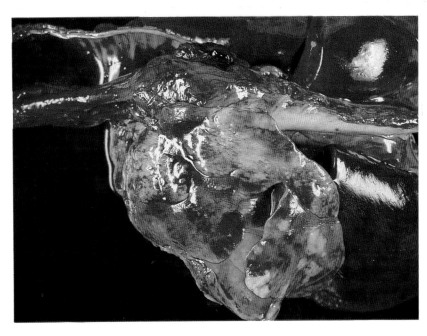

Plate 77 Choke

This dog entrapped a bone in the esophagus above the base of the heart.

II. Stenosis

Narrowing of the esophageal lumen occurs from compressive lesions caused by adjacent granulomas or tumors, from strictures and cicatrization as the result of a wound and as the result of congenital vascular ring anomalies.

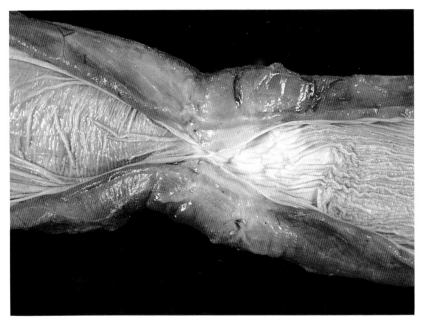

Plate 78 Stricture

Adhesions of traumatized mucosa leading to severe focal narrowing in the esophagus of this horse.

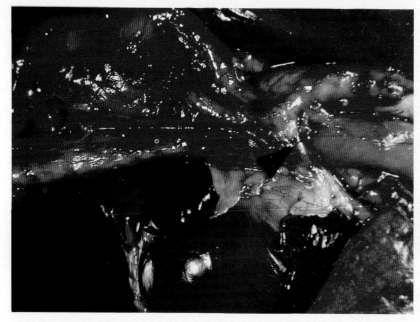

Plate 79 Vascular Ring Anomaly

If the fourth right aortic arch persists during the embryologic development of the aorta instead of the fourth left, which normally becomes the aorta, the ductus arteriosus and in the neonate the ligamentum arteriosum cross over the esophagus from the right side of the midline to the left constricting the esophagus and in advanced cases also the trachea. The constriction leads to megaesophagus starting cranial to the site of compression as depicted in this young dog.

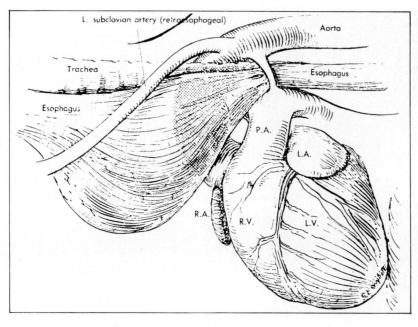

Plate 80 Megaesophagus Resulting from Vascular Ring Anomaly

Schematic drawing of site of constriction.

III. Perforation

Foreign bodies, wounds, chemicals or improper instrumentation lead to perforation of the esophageal wall with serious phlegmonous and gangrenous periesophageal inflammations which, in extreme cases, may develop into pleuritis or tracheo-esophageal fistulas.

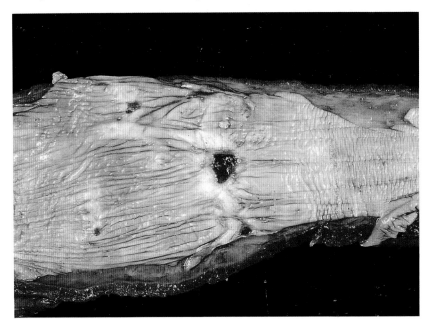

Plate 81 Perforation

Esophageal perforation in a horse which occurred during the passing of a stomach tube.

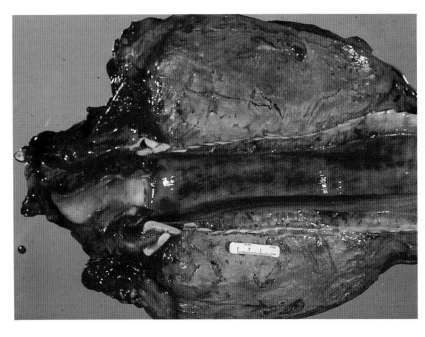

Plate 82 Perforation

Cervical phlegmon in a cow as a result of esophageal perforation from inappropriate deworming procedure.

IV. Dilatation and Achalasia

Sac-like dilatations which are unilateral and asymmetrical are referred to as diverticula. They are of two types - pulsion and traction. Pulsion diverticula are, more accurately, mucosal herniations through defects and tears in the muscularis. Traction diverticula result when periesophageal inflammation exerts traction on segments of the wall. Ectasia describes a uniform, symmetric dilatation of the esophageal wall and may be proximal to a point of stenosis. Achalasia means "failure to relax after swallowing" and leads to megaesophagus with dysphagia for both solids and liquids. Megaesophagus is frequently congenital but may be acquired and occurs principally in dogs. Three types have been described: cricopharyngeal, vascular ring anomalies and idiopathic megaesophagus affecting the entire length of the esophagus. It is presently believed that idiopathic megaesophagus in the dog is caused by neither cardiac sphincter failure nor by decreased numbers of intramural myenteric ganglion cells but by a motor abnormality of the nucleus ambiguus in the brain stem. These motor nuclei are responsible for the direct innervation of the esophagus in the dog.

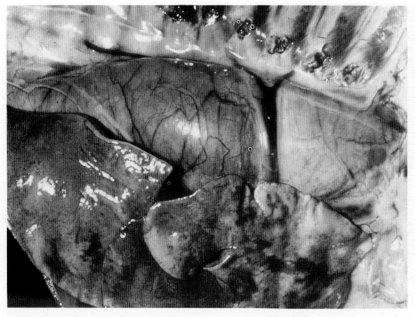

Plate 83 Idiopathic Megaesophagus

Idiopathic megaesophagus in a young dog. Note diffuse dilatation of the entire thoracic esophagus. Aspiration pneumonia is a common serious consequence of the disorder.

V. Inflammation

The specific viral diseases leading to inflammation of the esophageal mucosa have been discussed under " Inflammation of the Oral Cavity." They have to be differentiated from inflammatory processes caused by corrosive chemicals or thermal burns. Reflux esophagitis of the distal esophagus in dogs, horses and pigs is associated with protracted vomiting and spill-over of gastric contents into the esophagus. The basic defect for this disorder is incompetency of the lower esophageal sphincter (hypotonia). Debilitating diseases may lead to secondary infection with Candida albicans (thrush) in young nursing animals. This yeast organism produces concurrent lesions on the oral mucosa, the tongue and in the pharynx.

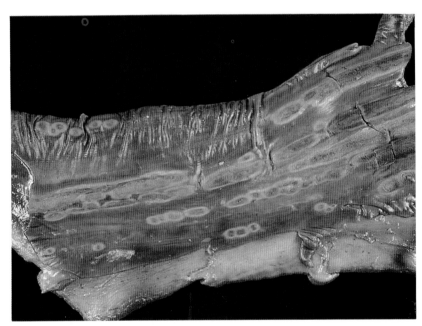

Plate 84 Erosions

Chronic corrosive scabby esophagitis in a cow. The severity depends on the nature of the chemical, its concentration and the duration of its contact with the mucosa. The raised plaques in the esophageal mucosa have to be differentiated from excessive keratinization and from ingestion of chlorinated naphthalenes.

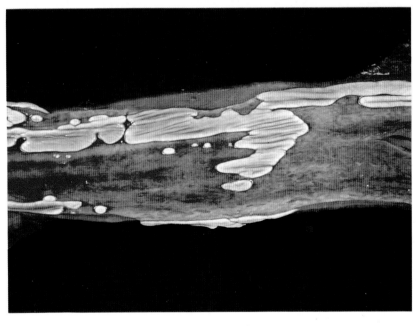

Plate 85 Erosions and Hyperkeratosis

Gastroduodenal ulcer disease has been recognized as important equine disorder in many countries. The disease is mainly recognized in foals and can co-exist with severe esophageal erosions and ulcerations. Much of the esophageal mucosa in this foal's esophagus has been lost while remaining mucosal islands have undergone hyperkeratinization. The denuded raw surface reacts with severe hyperemia and hemorrhage. Colonization with Candida sp. may be a secondary complication.

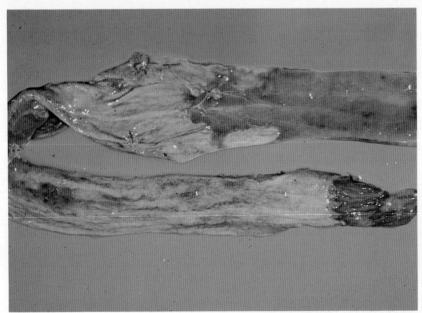

Plate 86 Reflux Esophagitis

Spill-over of gastric acids and bile re-sults in esophageal burns as present in this horse. Odynophagia is a clinical sign.

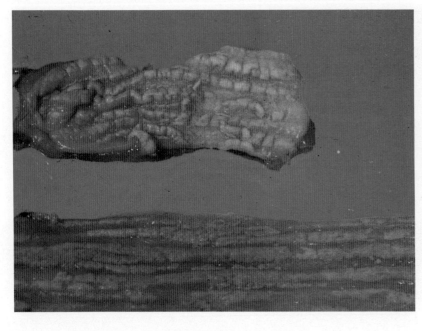

Plate 87 Candidiasis ("Thrush"; "Moniliasis")

Candida becomes a pathogen to the strat-ified squamous epithelium of the upper alimentary tract when the resistance of the host has been lowered. Raised whitish, crusty keratin plaques appear on the epithelial surface. In the severe cases the mucosal surface is encrusted with dry necrotic material.

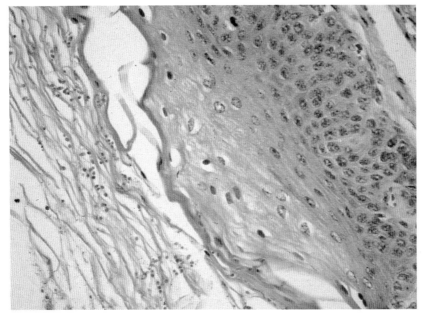

Plate 88 Candidiasis

Histologically, yeast and pseudohyphae of Candida make up the dry raised material. They are entangled in excess keratin. Inflammatory reactions are minimal. H&E stain.

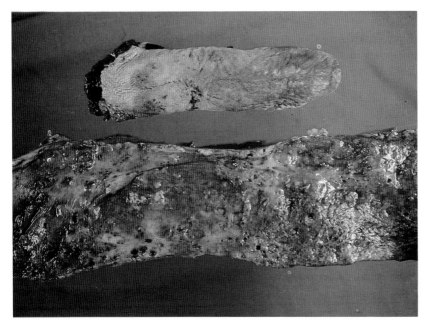

Plate 89 Pythiosis

Alimentary infection with Pythium has become an insidious disease in dogs kept in subtropical and tropical areas. Pythium insidiosum may invade any segment of the gastrointestinal tract to cause a deep, invasive, transmural necrogranulomatous inflammation. This young dog's tongue and esophagus are affected with pythiosis. The organisms extend into the stomach, large intestine and mesenteric lymph nodes.

VI. Parasitic Disease

Sarcosporidiosis in ruminants and horses.

Gasterophilus in the horse. Larvae of bots are occasionally attached to the mucosa of the distal esophagus.

Hypoderma lineatum in cattle. Larvae are lodged within the submucosa and the serosa.

Canine Spirocerca lupi. Adult worm nodules in the wall of the esophagus connect via fistulous tracts with the lumen.

Gongylonema in ruminants. Worms lodge in the superficial mucosa.

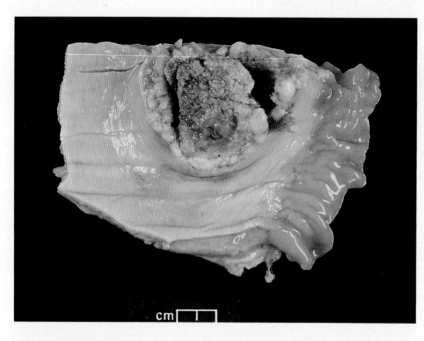

Plate 90   Spirocercosis

Spirocerca lupi in canine esophageal wall. Through fistulas communicating with the esophageal lumen, eggs are eliminated into the digestive tract. Occasionally the inflammatory nodes in the wall of the esophagus are transformed into malignant cells with fibrosarcomas and osteogenic sarcomas developing as in this case. After the third stage, infective larvae of Spirocerca lupi are ingested by the definitive host, penetrate the gastric mucosa and migrate up the gastric and gastric-epiploic arteries to the aorta where they concentrate in the wall of the thoracic aorta. From here they pass to the wall of the esophagus, either via the connective tissue or walls of the small arteries. Parasitic cysts and nodules develop in the wall of the esophagus.

Plate 91   Hypoderma lineatum or bovis

Larval migration tracts leave foci of hemorrhage, abscesses or fibrous scars on serosal surface of the bovine esophagus.

Larvae migrate on way to dermis of the back in cattle.

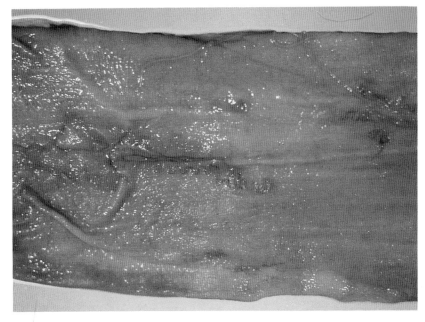

Plate 92　Gongylonemiasis

Thin, serpentine Gongylonema parasites lodge in the epithelium of a deer esophagus. The parasites do not evoke inflammatory responses and usually are incidental findings.

VII.　Neoplasms

Tumors of the esophagus are extremely rare in domestic animals. They sometimes occur in cats or horses as carcinomas or as lymphosarcomas in cattle.

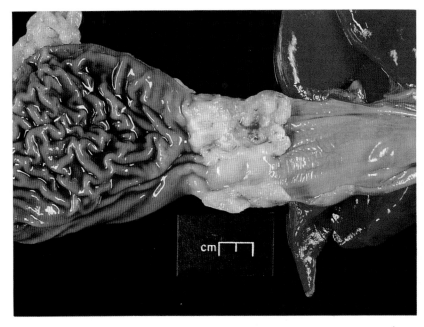

Plate 93　Feline Squamous Cell Carcinoma

The distal esophagus is obstructed by a sessile, white, nodular growth that extends into the cardia. Preceding esophagus segment is dilated.

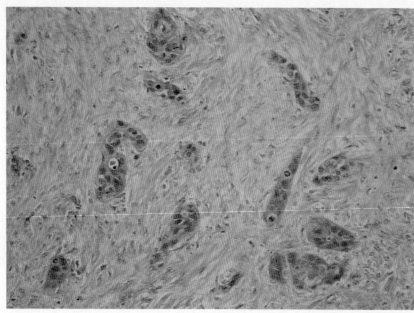

Plate 94   Feline Squamous Cell Carcinoma

Histologically, neoplastic squamous cells have invaded the esophagus wall to form keratin pearls and desmoplasia.   H&E stain.

VIII. Miscellaneous

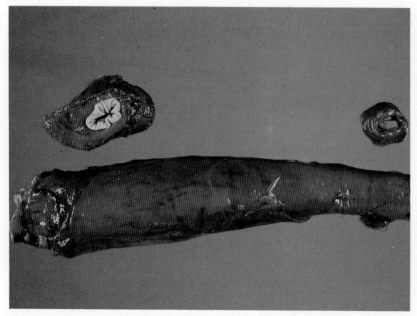

Plate 95   Idiopathic Esophageal Hypertrophy in the Horse

Many older horses reveal a thickening of the muscularis of the distal esophagus without functional complications.   The cause is unknown.

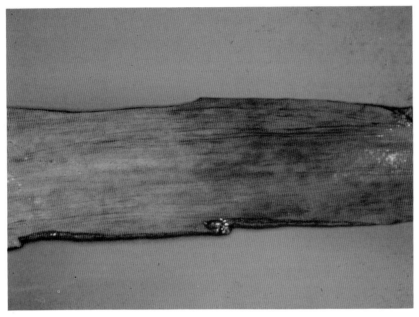

Plate 96   Bloat "Line"

Some cases of bovine tympany are associated with a line of purple-blue discoloration of the cranial esophagus mucosa definitively strengthening the diagnosis of antemortem bloat. It is the result of an ever distending rumen which compresses mainly blood-returning veins to cause vascular ischemia of the compressed segments and passive congestion of the peripheral segment.

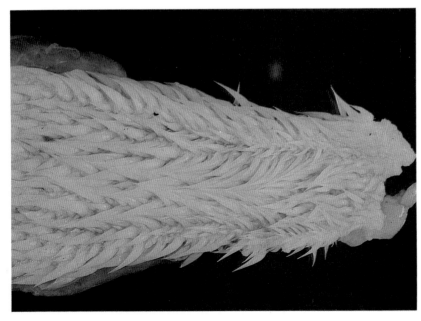

Plate 97   Esophagus of Sea Turtle

Horn-like papillae increase the absorption surface of the turtle esophagus and are normal structures. They should not be confused with papillomas.

Literature

1 . K.J. Whitehair, J.C. Cox, C.P. Coyne, R.M. DeBowes: Esophageal Obstruction in Horses. Comp. Cont. Ed. 12:91-96, 1990.

2 . T.L. Gross and I.G. Mayhew: Gastroesophageal Ulceration and Candidiasis in Foals. J. Am. Vet. Med. Assoc. 182:1370, 1983.

3 . P.C. Stromberg, K.A. Schwinghammer: Esophageal Gangylonemiasis in Cattle. Vet. Path. 25:241, 1988.

Chapter 3   Forestomachs and Stomach

A. The Ruminant Forestomachs
I. Dilatation of the Rumen

The accumulation of excessive quantities of gas - methane, CO_2, CO, H_2S and others - leads to ruminal distention also known as tympany or bloat. Bloat is the result of any interference with normal eructation (reflux spasms) or of the production of gas at a rate beyond the capacity of esophageal eructation to discharge it.

(a) Primary Tympany

Occurs acutely in cattle kept in feedlots or pastured on legumes. The excessive formation of fermentative gases and the inhibition of ruminal movement by toxic substances lead to either "free gas" or "frothy ingesta" types of bloat. Death is due to anoxia or dyspnea.

(b) Secondary Tympany

Physical (choke) or functional defects (tumors, vagal indigestion, adhesions) in the eructation of gases produced by normal fermentation lead to intermittent or chronic tympany. The postmortem findings are the same as for primar tympany.

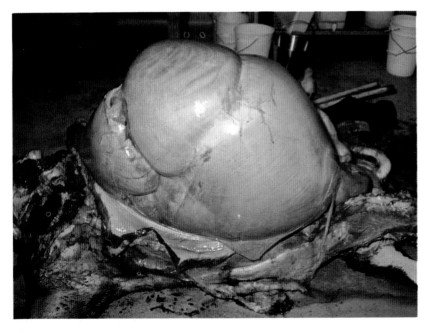

Plate 98   Tympany

In-situ appearance of bloat.

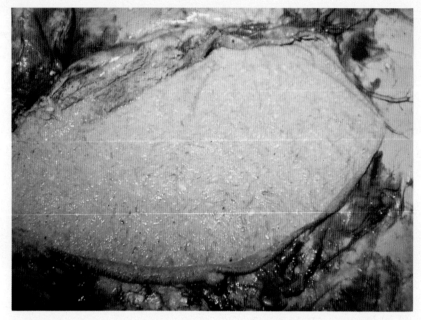

Plates 99   Frothy Tympany

Examples of "frothy" bloat in a cow.

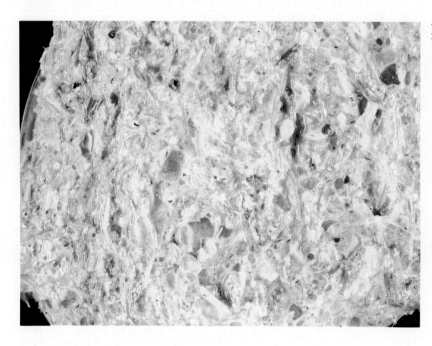

Plate 100   Frothy Tympany

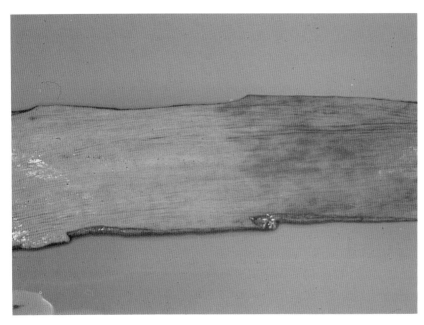

Plate 101   Bloat "Line"

The bloat "line" in the esophagus is a good indicator for acute antemortem tympany. The line demarcates a congested cranial esophageal mucosa from its pale caudal portion.

II.   Ruminal Atony

Vagal paralysis interferes with ruminal contraction and leads to impaction and intoxication. Omasal and abomasal impactions occur.

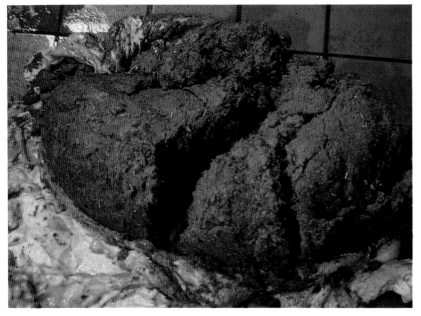

Plate 102 Impaction.

This is ruminal impaction. Ingesta are dry, hardened.

III. Metabolic Disorders
Ruminal Acidosis

Life-threatening disorder. also known as "overeating" disease or acute acid indigestion. Food rich in carbo-hydrates produces excessive amounts of lactic acid which drops the pH of the rumen as low as 4.0. Many bac-teria of the normal ruminal flora are killed by the low pH.Lactobacilli and Streptococcus lactis continue to proliferate as the ruminal pH changes. and atony of the rumen develops. Increased lactate causes metabolic acidosis. It also increases ruminal osmotic pressure with sodium and body fluids being drawn into the rumen resulting in dehydration. hypovolemia and hemoconcentration.Circulatory collapse is the cause of death.

Opportunistic agents are responsible for infective complications in overeating disease. These are commonly either Fusobacterium necrophorum (necrobacillary rumenitis) or Mucor sp. (mucormycotic rumenitis). The organisms cause ruminal ulcers and spread into the liver where necrosis and abscesses develop.

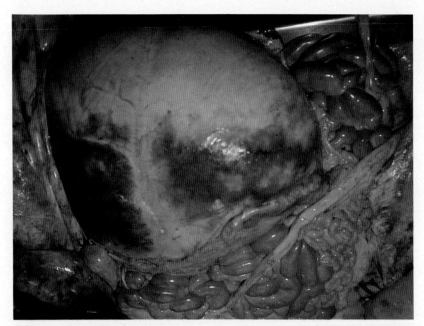

Plate 103   Acid Indigestion

"Overeating" disease as characterized by red-brown transmural discolorations of the rumen.

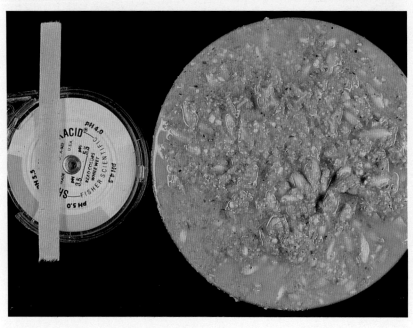

Plate 104   Acid Indigestion

Checking the pH for evidence of exces-sive lactic acid.

IV. Inflammations

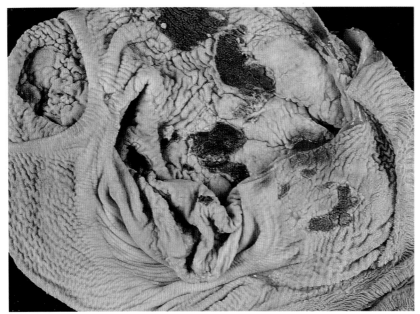

Plate 105 Mycotic Rumenitis

Button ulcers with well demarcated, elevated margins are characteristic findings in the mucosa secondary to acid indigestion.

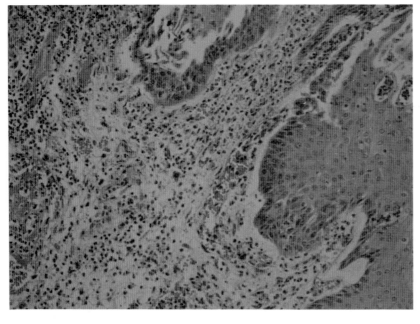

Plate 106 Mycotic Rumenitis

Invasion of fungi into submucosal blood vessels with vascular thrombosis is responsible for rumen ulceration. H&E stain.

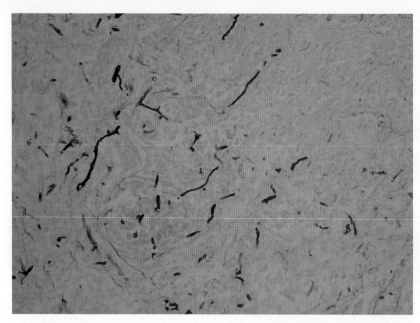

Plate 107 Mycotic Rumenitis

Mycelia of fungus in mycotic rumenitis. These usually belong to Aspergillus sp. or to Mucor sp. such as Absidia and Rhizopus. GMS stain.

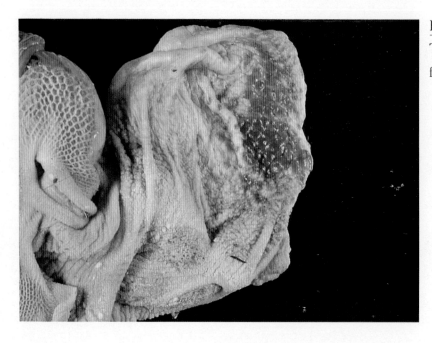

Plate 108 Mycotic Rumenitis

This young calf's ruminal mucosa is diffusely reddened.

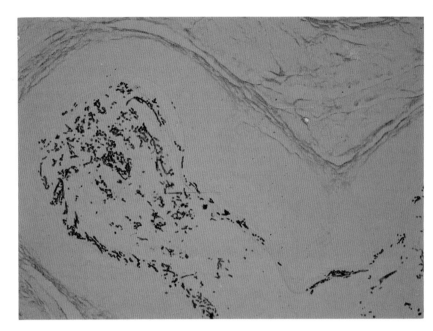

Plate 109 Mycotic Rumenitis

Histologically, the mucosal surface is colonized by yeasts and pseudomycelia of Candida sp. GMS stain.

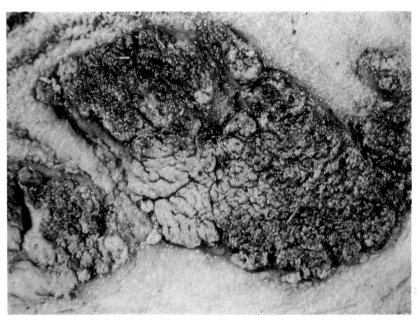

Plate 110   Necrobacillary Rumenitis

Multiple, irregular, elevated, slightly necrotic plaques and scabs are spread throughout the mucosa. Hepatic "metastases" are frequently associated with ruminal necrobacillosis (Fusobacterium necrophorum).

Plate 111   Toxic Rumenitis

Acute lead poisoning in a cow after ingestion of excessive amounts of crankcase
oil. Note the oil slick on the floor.

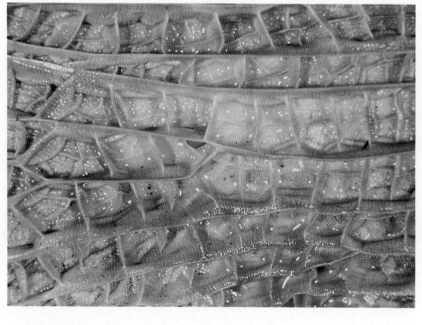

Plate 112   Traumatic Reticu-
loperitonitis

Traumatic reticuloperitonitis in cattle
caused by nails or wires leads to local
abscesses in the reticulum or perforation
of the reticular wall with focal or chronic extensive peritonitis and pericarditis.
Pyogenic bacteria commonly involved are
Actinomyces pyogenes, Pseudomonas aeruginosa and Fusobacterium necrophorum.

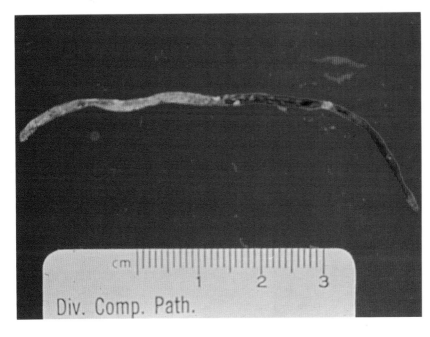

Div. Comp. Path.

Plate 113 Traumatic Reticulitis

Loose, sharp foreign bodies of more than 5 cm length penetrate through the reticulum to create a fistulous tract and septic peritonitis. They slowly may move through the diaphragm towards the pericardial sac.

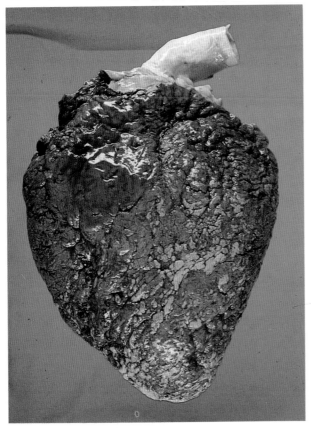

Plate 114 Traumatic Pericarditis

As pyogenic bacteria are carried into the pericardial sac, cor villosum or "shaggy heart" disease develops. The pericardium of such heart is covered with a thick layer of white and yellow fibrin. Free seropurulent exudate distends the pericardial sac and causes adhesions to induce constrictive pericarditis.

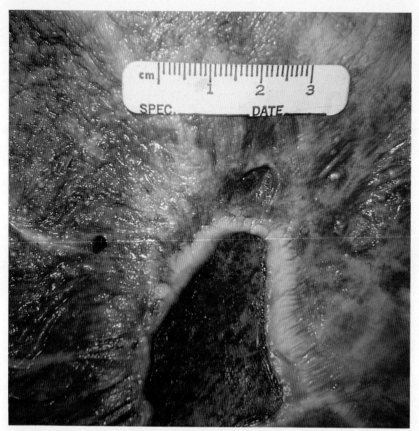

Plates 115, 116   Ruminal Scars

Chronic ruminal ulcers associated with hardware disease. These ulcers healed uneventfully. They also should be considered as being the end result of transient acid indigestion.

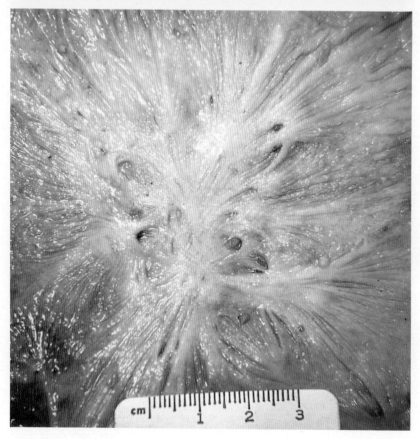

Plate 116   Ruminal Scars

Urea Poisoning

This non-protein, nitrogen feed supplement may be fed in too high a concentration as the result of mixing errors. It becomes toxic if it represents more than 3% of the feed mixture.

$$\text{Nitrogen} \xrightarrow[\text{urease}]{\text{ruminal}} NH_3 + CO_2$$

V. Endoparasites

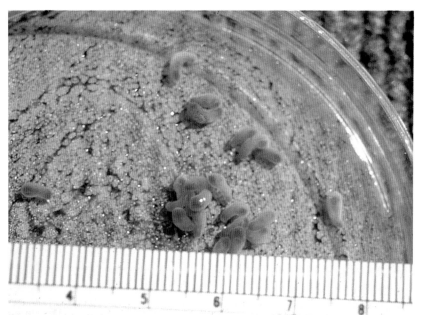

Plate 117   Ruminal Flukes

The conical, reddish, droplet-shaped flukes are ruminal parasites and usually non-pathogenic. Flukes of the genus Paramphistomum inhabit the reticulum and rumen. Although there are reports of mortality associated with these parasites, they are generally considered harmless. Only heavy infestation causes diarrhea, rapid weight loss and anemia due to the presence of larval forms in the duodenum. Because they are flesh-colored, they are easily overlooked on "casual" examination of the rumen.

VI. Neoplasms

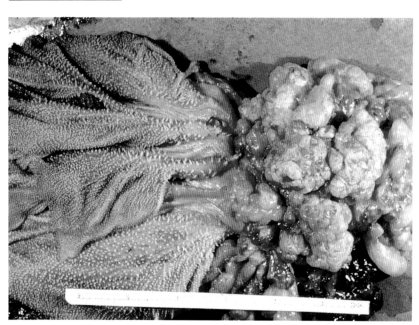

Plate 118   Papilloma

Benign papillomas develop in all compartments, but are more common in the reticulum. Malignant lymphomas occasionally involve the forestomach.

B. The Stomach

Major gastric functions are (1) storage of large quantities of food until it can be accommodated in the lower portion of the gastrointestinal tract. (2)mixing of food with gastric secretions and (3) slow emptying of food from the stomach into the small intestine at a rate for proper digestion and absorption by the small intestine.

The true stomach is divided into three regions: (1) esophageal region ‑ lined with stratified squamous epithelium in some animal species. e.g. swine. horse.   (2)glandular region ‑ a. gastric fundic glands secreting pepsin by chief cells and hydrochloric acid by parietal cells.   b. pyloric glands secreting mucus. (3) antrum. Little absorption takes place in the stomach.   Only a few highly lipid soluble substances such as alcohol and some drugs are absorbed.

I. Changes in Position

Acute Dilatation and Volvulus Complex

Gastric displacement occurs primarily in cattle. dogs. monkeys and rabbits. Fermentable feed. air from suction (aerophagia) and replicating anaerobes are suggested as precipitating factors.   Bloat. rotation and rupture are pathologic consequences.   The following is offered as general definitions for gastrointestinal displacements (rotations):

(a) **Volvulus: Twist of hollow organ around the axis of its suspension (mesentery).**

(b) **Torsion: Twist of hollow organ around its own longitudinal axis.**

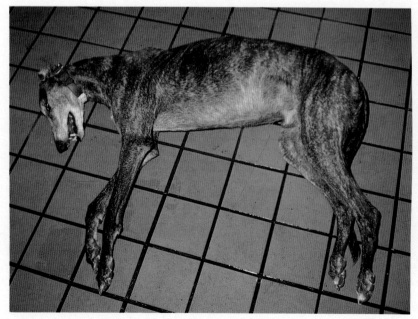

Plate 119   Acute Gastric Dilatation (AGD)

The abdominal cavity is distended by the stomach in a case of acute gastric dilatation.   The enlarged stomach has moved from its usual left position in the abdomen to a craniocaudal longitudinal position.

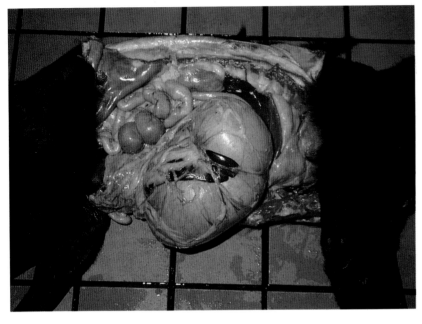

Plate 120 Gastric Volvulus

Dog with acute gastric dilatation, compli-
cated by volvulus, shows an enlarged
stomach, which has stretched on its
greater curvature and has twisted around
its mesenteric axis. The spleen has
moved with the rotating stomach from
the left to the right side coming to rest
against the right diaphragm, folded tight-
ly in a "V" by its taut gastrosplenic ligament. The omentum partially drapes the
stomach. The gastric volvulus is 270
degrees, clockwise.

Bacterial cultivation of stomach contents
from animals with AGD may result in
some isolation of anaerobes and Bacillus
sp. and less of gram-negative bacteria
when compared with the stomach contents of normal dogs. Clinically gastric
distention quickly leads to tissue acidosis,
cardiac arrhythmias,disseminated intravas-
cular coagulation, hypotension and cardio-
genic shock.Death ensues if treatment is
delayed or inadequate. The AGD complex
is seen predominantly in large or giant
breed, deep chested dogs such as German
Shepherd dogs, Great Danes, Irish Set-
ters, Doberman Pinshers, Saint Bernard
dogs .

Plate 121 Gastric Eversion

Portion of the cranial stomach has tele-
scoped into the distal esophagus causing
marked distention and stenosis.

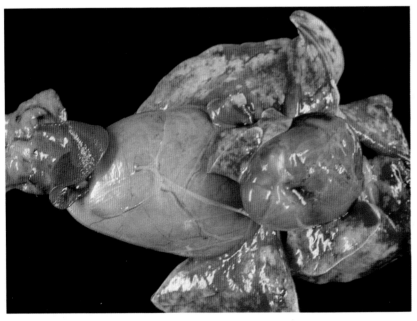

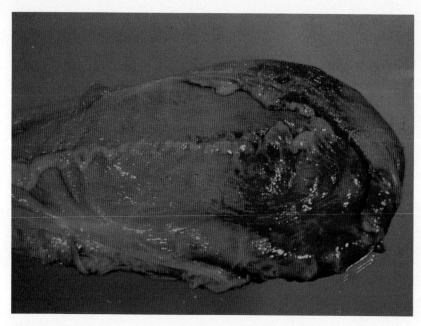

Plate 122   Gastric Eversion

The herniated segment of the stomach is characterized by transmural serosal congestion and hemorrhage.

Displacement of the Abomasum in Cattle

In this condition the abomasum glides across the abdominal wall from right to left into a left-sided dislocation.It rests between the rumen and abdominal wall. Results are atony with dilatation and gas accumulation. Cases peak in March and April. Displacement may occur immediately following parturition.with hypocalcemia resulting from high lactation or ketosis or after high concentrate feeding with increased volatile fatty acid production. Left and right-sided displacements have been described; the ratio is 5:1. Hypochloremia and metabolic alkalosis are clinicopathologic consequences.

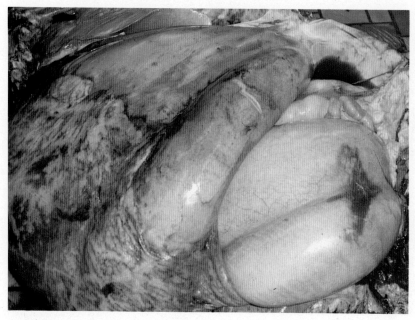

Plate 123 Left-sided Abomasal Displacement

The abomasal displacement resulted from a 90 degree counter-clockwise rotation around its vertical axis. Fatal consequences are necrosis. peritonitis or rupture due to pyloris stenosis or impaction.

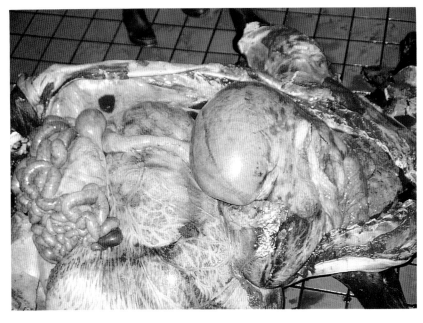

Plate 124 Right-sided Abomasal Displacement

The abomasum has rotated upwards and cranial on the right side. It is extremely gas-filled.

II. Gastric Dilatation and Rupture in the Horse

This condition always occurs at the greater curvature. The majority of the cases are idiopathic, others are the result of intestinal obstruction, ileus or overeating of grass/ alfalfa hay coupled with gastric overdistention. Gastric displacement does not take place.

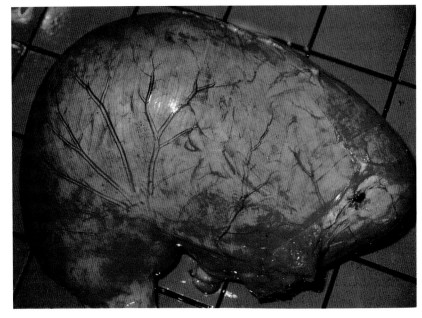

Plates 125-128 Gastric Rupture

Rupture of distended equine stomach. The serosa is dissected from the muscularis. Edges are rugged, swollen and hemorrhagic. Death often occurs before there is time for peritonitis to develop. It is due to shock or due to hemorrhage.

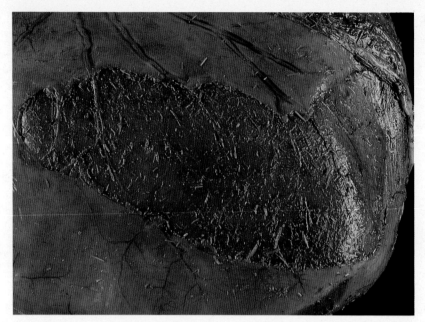

Plate 126   Gastric Rupture

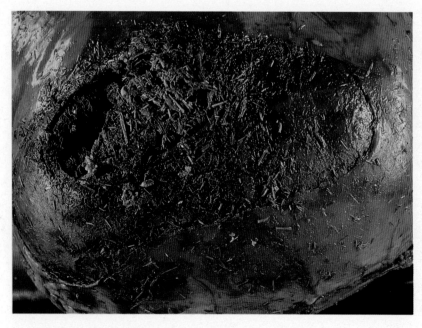

Plate 127   Gastric Rupture

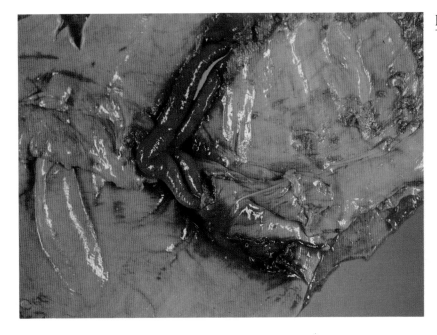

Plate 128   Gastric Rupture

III.   Foreign Bodies

Hairballs (trichobezoars) or plant fiber balls (phytobezoars) are common in young animals.   They usually do not interfere with ruminal function and are incidental findings.

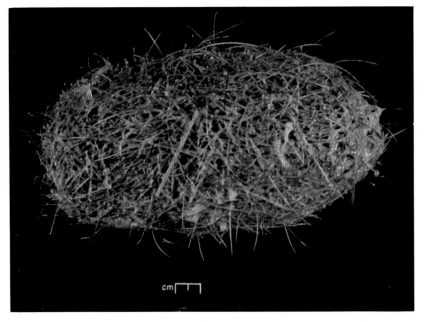

Plate 129   Hairball

Phytobezoar from within stomach of pig.

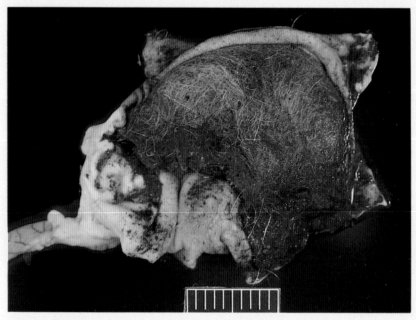

Plate 130   Hairball

Hairball from rabbit stomach. The hair-ball may extend the stomach to rupture and to cause sudden death. The condition is a management problem in laboratory rabbit colonies.

IV.   Gastric Ulcers

Ulcerations represent a circumscribed break in areas of the gastric mucosa which is normally bathed by hydrochloric acid and pepsin. The breaks may be superficial or deep. Mucosal breaks which do not penetrate below the lamina muscularis mucosae are erosions. Ulcers penetrate below the lamina muscularis mucosae. Acute ulcers do not manifest a fibrous tissue response. Chronic ulcers demonstrate a significant fibrous tissue response.

Causes : a. mechanic d. mycotic
    b. toxic   e. neoplastic
    c. dietary   f. drug-induced

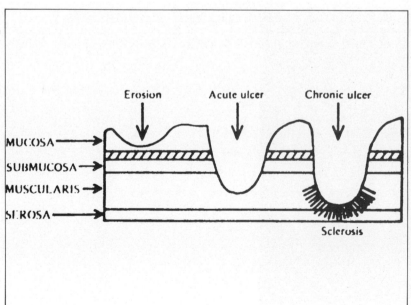

Plate 131   Gastric Erosions and Ulcers

Schematic diagrams illustrating the degree of mucosal breaks.

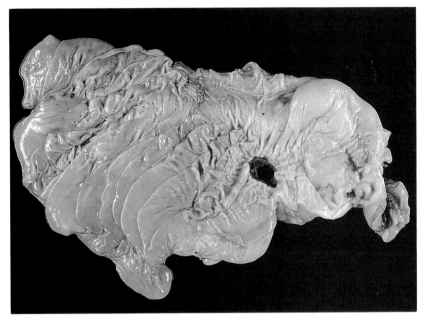

Plate 132　Peptic Ulcer

Hyperacidity from sudden changes from soft to rough feed has been accused of causing gastric ulcers present in calves in the first three months of life. They usually involve the pyloric mucosa near its junction.　Some ulcers perforate.

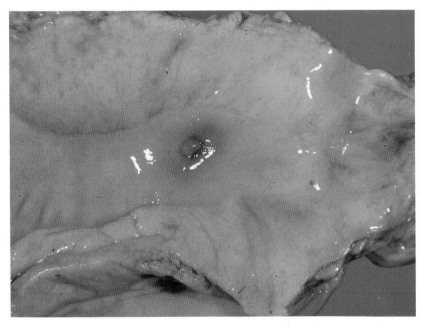

Plate 133　Perforating Ulcer

Perforating ulcers in adult cattle may be associated with foreign bodies causing pyloric obstruction, calving and lactation. Ulcer edges are sharp, punched-out.

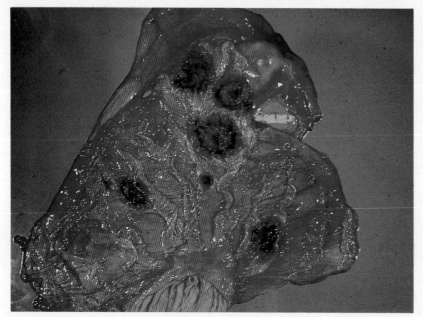

Plate 134 Mycotic Ulcer

Mycotic ulcers occur in situations of debilitating infections or excessive antibiotic therapy. Note the elevated edges and the central necrotic,hemorrhagic exudate on the surface of the ulcers in this calf's abomasum.

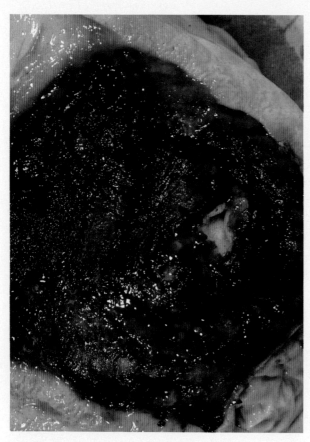

Plate 135 Bleeding Ulcer

Ulcers of dietary (finely ground rations) or stress origin in weaned feeder pigs are confined to the pars esophagea. The squamous mucosa can be ulcerated in its entirety. Death usually occurs promptly from massive gastric hemorrhage. The cadaver is anemic. Dark, tarry stool is passed through the intestinal tract (melena).

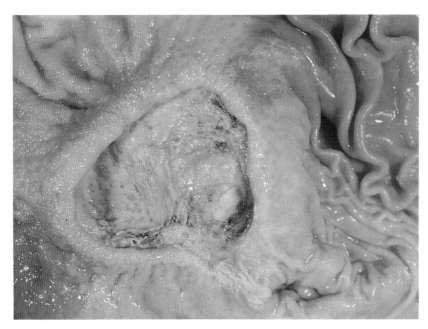

Plate 136   Chronic Ulcer
The ulcer edge is very prominent, and most of the central portion of the ulcer is denuded squamous cell lining.

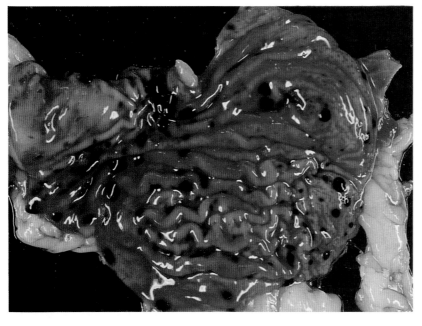

Plate 137   Gastric Erosions
This is an example of drug-induced erosions and bleeding in a canine stomach. This dog was treated with steroids. Prolonged aspirin treatment or consumption can cause small bleeding erosions as well.

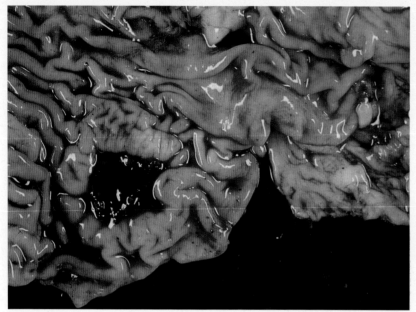

Plates 138,139   Bleeding Ulcer

Ulcerations in the mucosa of the gastric pylorus or of the duodenum in cats and dogs may be associated with dermal or visceral mast cell tumors. The ulcers are believed to be caused by the effect of biogenic amine release from the neoplastic cells.   The dog suffered from severe melena and is extremely anemic.

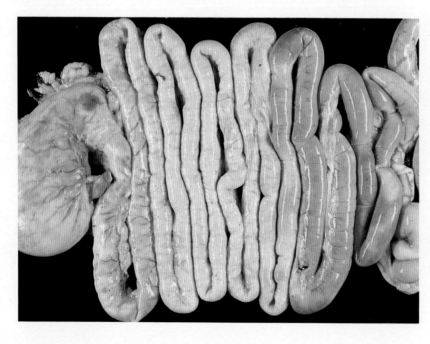

Plate 139   Bleeding Ulcer

V. Gastroduodenal Ulcers in Foals

Gastric ulceration became an important disease in foal rearing because an increasing number of foals developed signs of colic and died suddenly from perforated gastric or duodenal ulcers, the cause of which is probably multifactorial. Several hypotheses have been advanced, but few have been proven. Environmental stress such as heat, overcrowding and excessive handling have been associated with the disease. Excessive dosing with or susceptibility to the effects of nonsteroidal anti-inflammatory drugs (NSAID) have been incriminated as ulcerogenic as have been indigenous steroids secreted into the milk of highly lactating mares. Likewise, dietary factors are believed to play a role in the cause of the disease. The pathophysiology of gastroduodenal ulceration remains poorly understood. Studies indicated that the prevalence of the lesions is greatest in foals below 10 days of age.

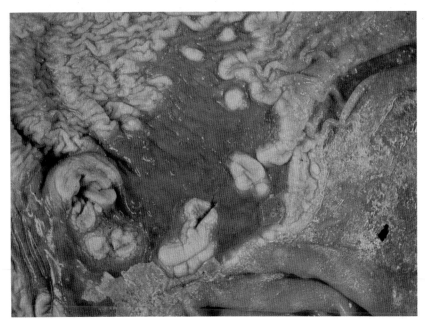

Plates 140,141 Gastric Erosions and Perforating Ulcers

Erosions and ulcers may either occur in the squamous cell portion of the foal stomach as shallow but extensive breaks or in the gastric mucosa as clearly delineated mucosal breaks which frequently lead to perforations.

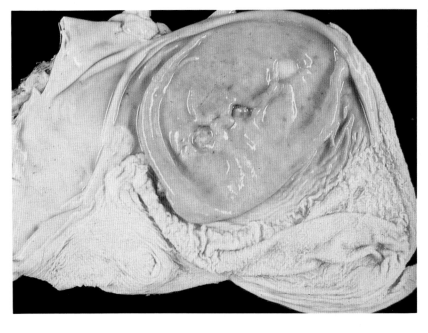

Plate 141 Gastric Erosions and Perforating Ulcers

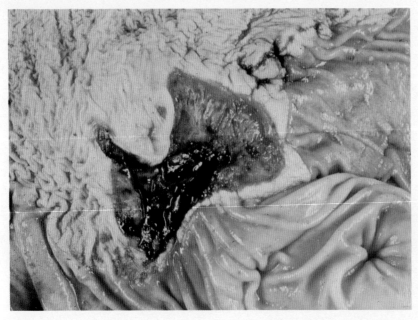

Plates 142, 143   Bleeding Ulcer

In some instances, bleeding ulcers occur with melena. These changes have been attributed to treatment with nonsteroidal, anti-inflammatory drugs such as phenyl-butazone and benamine. The ulcers also occur in the stomach of adult horses and are thought to be due to a toxic side effect of the drug on the gastric microcirculation and due to the effacement of the cytoprotective effects of prostaglandins.

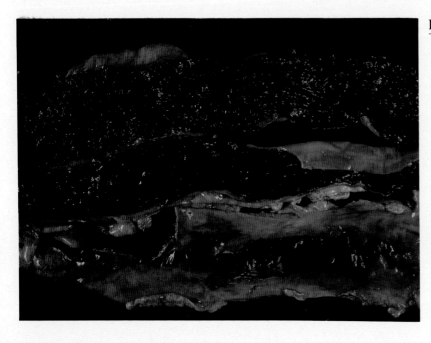

Plate 143   Bleeding Ulcer

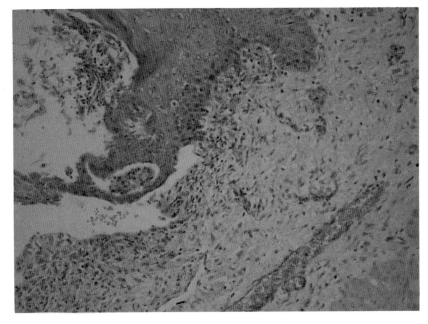

Plates 144, 145 Gastric Ulceration

Histologically, sequestration of the mucosal layer and denudation of the entire surface becomes evident. Other than extravasation and occasional thrombosis, very little inflammation is present. The occasional colonization with Candida is secondary to opportunistic invasion of the yeast. H&E, PAS stains.

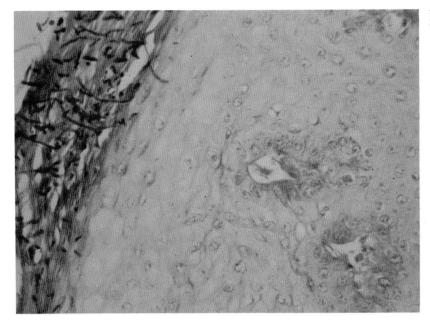

Plate 145 Gastric Ulceration

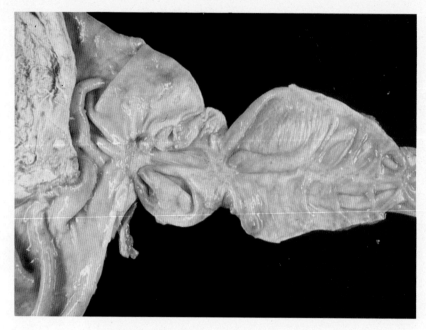

Plate 146   Chronic Ulcers

Duodenal strictures are complications from healing attempts of the ulcers. Proximal duodenal obstruction becomes apparent.   Animals exhibit signs of restlessness, inappetence, bruxism, and excessive salivation.   In advanced cases, dehydration, hypochloremia and metabolic alkalosis can occur.

VI.   Inflammation
Gastritis

Many lesions of the stomach referred to as gastritis are not inflammatory. The discrepancy is in part due to an abuse of the term, but in part also to the lack of well-defined criteria of mucosal inflammation.

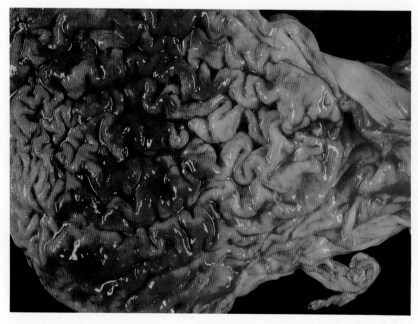

Plate 147   Acute Gastritis

In acute gastritis, the mucosa is hemorrhagic and edematous. Small erosions may be present.   Gastritis such as this may be associated with the ingestion of toxic substances, but may be also seen in infectious conditions and uremia.

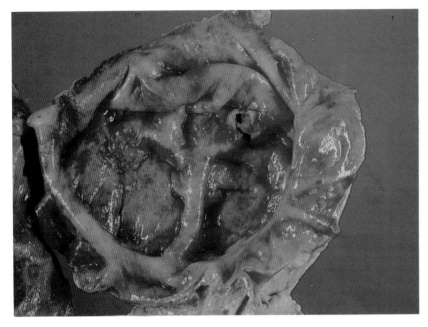

Plate 148 Uremic Gastritis

Gastric mucosa of an uremic horse. The mucosal folds are characterized by hemorrhage and mineralization.

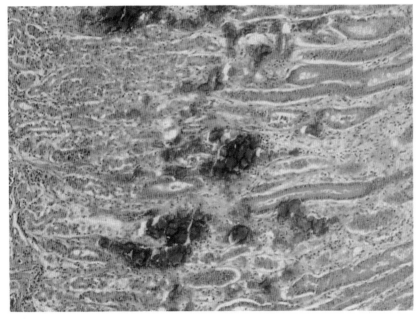

Plates 149, 150 Uremic Gastritis

Microscopically, fibrinoid necrosis of medium-sized arteries is seen in the gastric submucosa with uremia as well as varying degrees of midzonal mineralization of the mucosa and hyperemia of the very superficial capillaries. Vasculitis may be due to the circulation of toxic peptides associated with uremia. H&E stain.

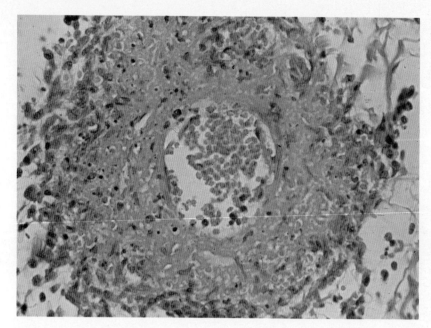

Plate 150 Uremic Gastritis

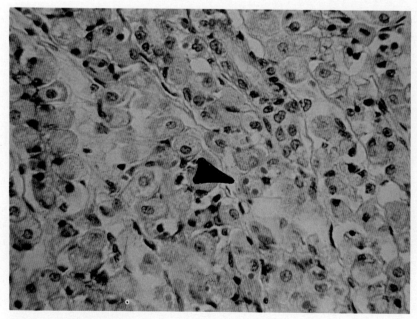

Plate 151 Canine Distemper

Canine distemper is seldom associated with gastritis. However, in cases of distemper infection, eosinophilic intracytoplasmic inclusion bodies are often found within the epithelial cells lining the crypts (arrow).

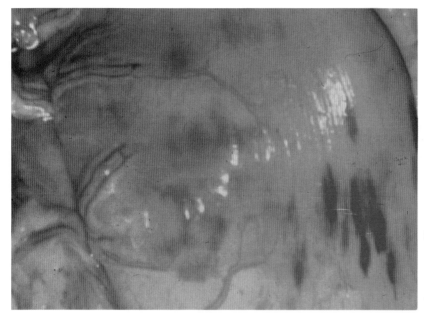

Plate 152 Canine Infectious Hepatitis

Paintbrush serosal hemorrhages of the stomach may be encountered in Canine Infectious Hepatitis.

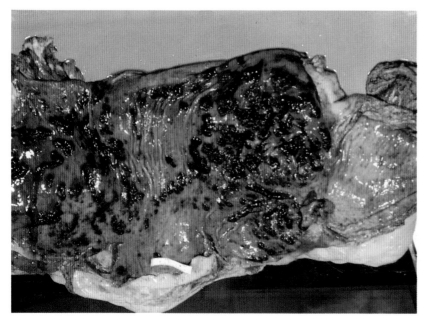

Plate 153 Toxic Abomasitis

This is the appearance of the mucosa of the abomasum of a cow with arsenic poisoning.

Differentials include corrosive chemicals, bleeding ulcers and infestation with Haemonchus contortus.

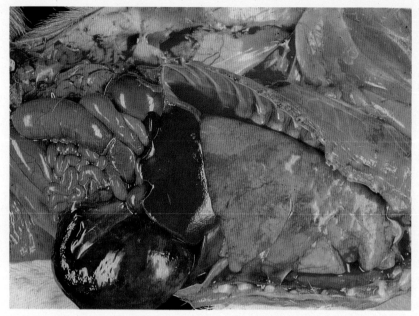

Plate 154   Braxy

Braxy of sheep is an acute hemorrhagic abomasitis caused by Clostridium septicum. It is largely a disease of lambs and yearling sheep following very cold weather. Once having invaded the tissues, the organisms elaborate exotoxins which are responsible for the clinical signs and death. The disease may occasionally affect calves.

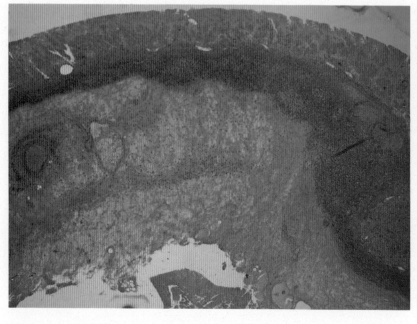

Plate 155   Braxy

Microscopically, the abomasum of braxy affected animals is characterized by mucosal hemorrhage and necrosis with peripheral neutrophilic demarcation as well as by edema and gas formation in the submucosa. H&E stain.

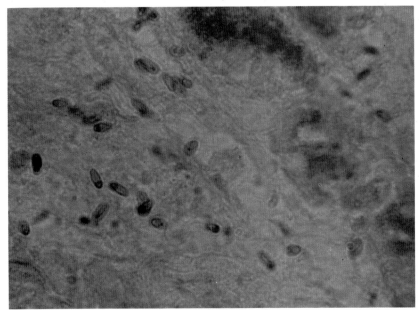

Plate 156 Braxy
Clostridial spores can be demonstrated within the lesion by GMS stains.

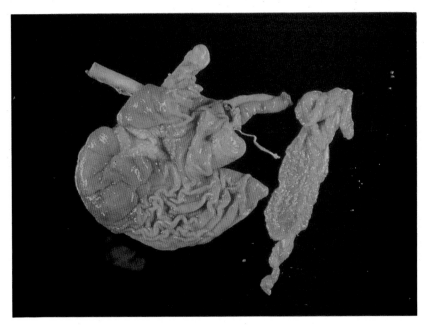

Plate 157 Edema Disease
This slide demonstrates Edema Disease in pigs. The edematous infiltration of the stomach wall is the result of generalized vasculitis caused by Shiga-like toxins elaborated by certain strains of E. coli. Typically, Edema Disease occurs in rapidly growing healthy animals between 4 and 8 weeks of age. The exact pathogenic mechanism has not been fully worked out, but there is evidence that the disease is an enterotoxemic colibacillosis with systemic involvement of the brain, subcutis, stomach, intestine, lung and pericardial sac.

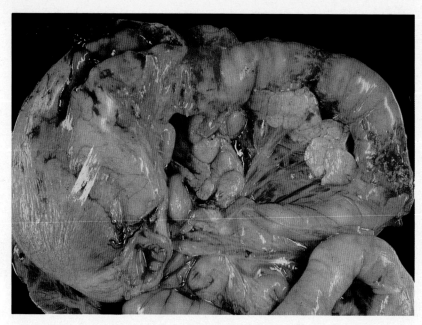

Plate 158 Pythiosis
A transmural necrohemorrhagic and proliferative inflammation mimicking a neoplasm is associated with invasive Pythium insidiosum infection in the canine alimentary tract. There is much extension into the surrounding serosal tissue including lymphadenopathy of draining lymph nodes.

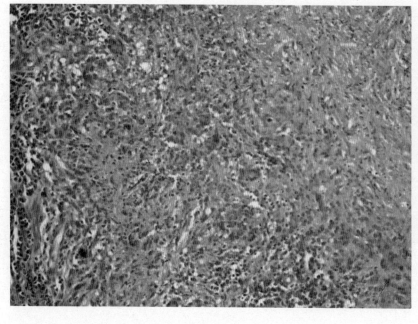

Plates 159, 160 Pythiosis
A necrotizing pyogranulomatous inflammatory response to the presence of invasive organisms is present at the microscopic level in pythiosis.The organism can be detected with special stains. Mucormycosis or infection with Zygomycetes has to be considered in the differential diagnosis. H&E, GMS stains.

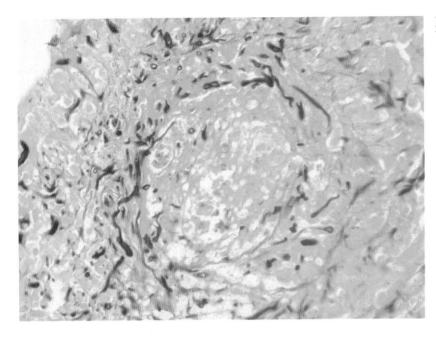

Plate 160 Pythiosis

VII. Endoparasites

Dogs and Cats: Physaloptera
Ollulanus tricuspis

Horses: Draschia megastoma
Habrenoma muscae
Habrenoma majus
Trichostrongylus axei
Gasterophilus sp.

Swine: Hyostrongylus rubidus
Ruminants: Haemonchus contortus
Ostertagia ostertagi
Trichostrongylus axei

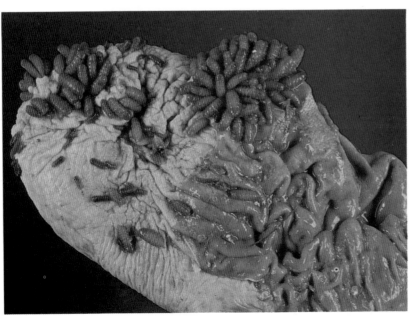

Plate 161 Gasterophilosis

Larvae of the bot flies of Gasterophilus sp. are found on the gastric mucosa of the horse. The larvae of G. intestinalis are the most common and attach themselves to the squamous region of the stomach. The larvae of G. nasalis are attached to the glandular mucosa near the pylorus. These attachments are usually of little consequence unless large numbers are present, in which case a gastritis with erosions and ulcers may result.

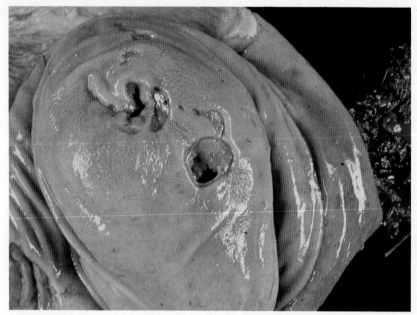

Plate 162 Habronemiasis

The adults of the equine parasite Draschia megastoma burrow into the gastric mucosa causing tumor-like inflammatory nodules, as shown here in the plicate margin. Squamous cell carcinoma should be considered as differential diagnosis.

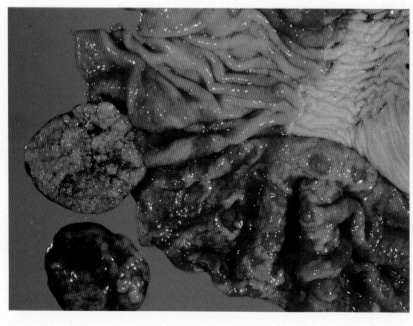

Plate 163 Trichostrongylosis

T. axei caused a chronic hyperplastic gastritis in this horse's stomach.

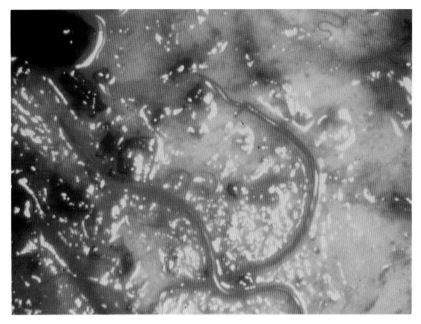

Plate 164   Haemonchosis

This is the abomasum of a sheep. Several Haemonchus sp. up to 2 cm long can be seen on the mucosa. The abomasal mucosa is hyperemic and shows blood spots or focal erosions at the points to which the parasites were attached. The life cycle is direct. The parasite is commonly referred to as "barberpole" worm.

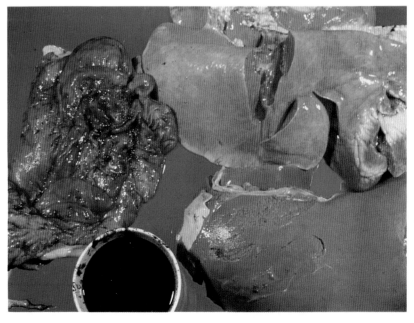

Plate 165   Haemonchosis

The worm is a blood sucker which commonly causes fatal anemia. Note the pallor of internal organs. Hypoproteinemia, "bottle jaw" due to subcutaneous edema and achlorhydria are additional clinical complications.

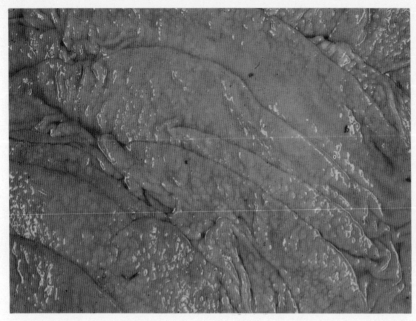

Plates 166,167   Ostertagiosis

Ostertagiosis is another important parasitic disease affecting ruminants. When
the larvae burrow into the mucosa, they
produce small, whitish, elevated nodules
in the abomasum due to epithelial metaplasia and hyperplasia. All of the abomasum may be involved in severe infestation. Hypoproteinemia,diarrhea, wasting
and death are major clinical complications.

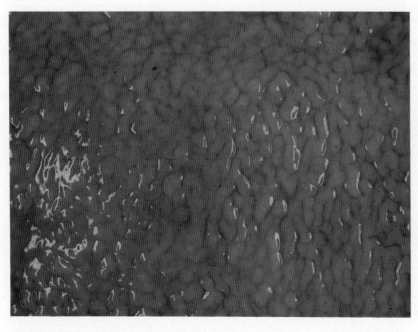

Plate   167   Ostertagiosis

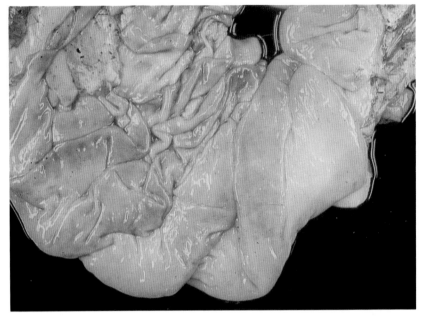

Plate 168   Ostertagiosis
Marked edema of abomasal folds suggests hypoproteinemia.

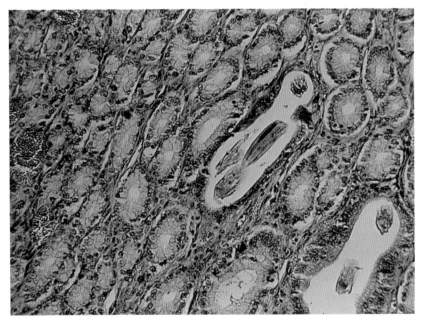

Plate 169 Ostertagiosis
Histologically, the larvae are present deep in the gastric pits and glands. They typically have longitudinal cuticular ridges on the surface.

VIII. Neoplasms

1. Carcinoma, sclerosing - horses and dogs.
2. Leiomyoma, leiomyosarcoma - dogs and cats.
3. Lymphoma - in cattle, dogs, cats, and pigs.
4. Neoplasms of the APUD - cell system (Amine precursor uptake and decarboxylation)

Special endocrine cells which process and secrete polypeptide hormones involved in digestion are scattered along the upper gut. These cells are of neural crest origin. They are fluorescent under formaldehyde vapors, stain metachromatically and stain positively with silver stains (argyrophilic). The cells may give rise to functional neoplasms (e.g. carcinoid tumors) in man, but little is known about them in animals. Occasionally, carcinoid tumors have been diagnosed in cats and dogs without follow-up study of their endocrinologic activities.

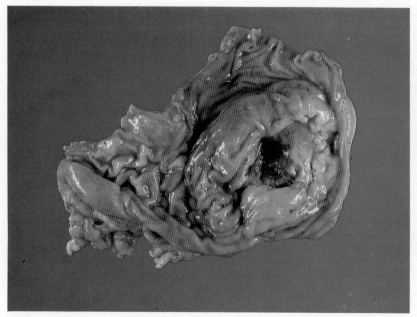

Plate 170 Gastric Adenocarcinoma

A fungating, ulcerative growth has replaced the normal gastric mucosa. The ulcer edges are irregular and crater-like. The central portion of the crater contains clotted blood. In the dog the tumors tend to arise from the lesser curvature of the stomach or the pylorus.

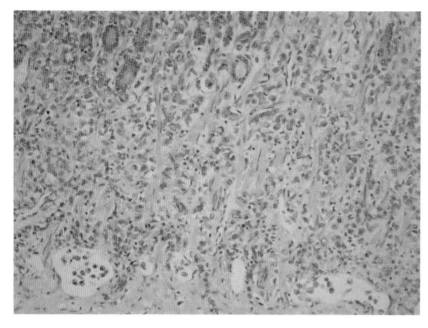

Plate 171   Gastric Adenocarcinoma

Histologically necrotic mucosal cells have invaded the gastric wall. Neoplastic cells form acini and tubules (intestinal type). Others are individualized or form sheets. Individual cells can be of signet-ring type containing mucus in the cytoplasm. Metastases first occur to regional lymph nodes.   H&E stain.

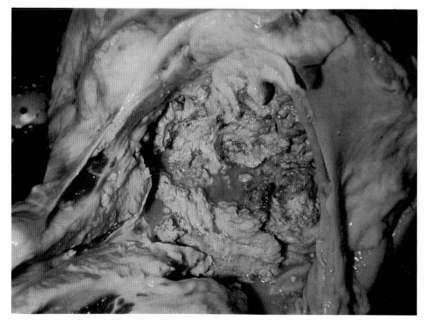

Plate 172   Gastric Squamous Cell Carcinoma

The lumen of the equine stomach has been filled with odoriferous, cauliflower, soft, necrotic tumor tissue which arises from the non-glandular part. The neoplastic cells invade the wall to disseminate on to the serosa and within the peritoneal cavity.

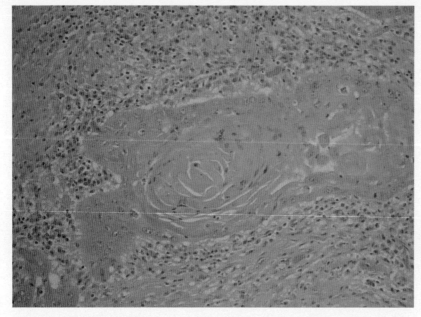

Plate 173 Gastric Squamous Cell Carcinoma

Typically, the microscopic appearance of the neoplasms is characterized by islands of neoplastic squamous cells forming keratin pearls and inciting a desmoplastic reaction. H&E stain.

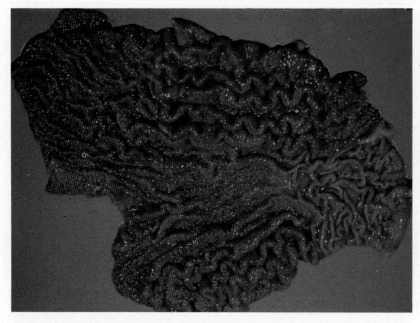

Plate 174 Gastric Lymphosarcoma

Mucosal folds are diffusely thickened in the dog's stomach. In cats, lymphosarcomas are more nodular and bulging. Lymphosarcomas of the alimentary tract account for 5% to 7% of all canine lymphosarcomas.

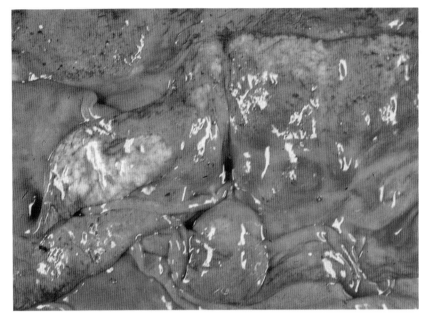

Plates 175, 176 Abomasal Lymphosarcoma

Abomasal folds are distended and thickened by white, fish-meat-like soft plaques. Neoplastic ulcers are frequent secondary complications.

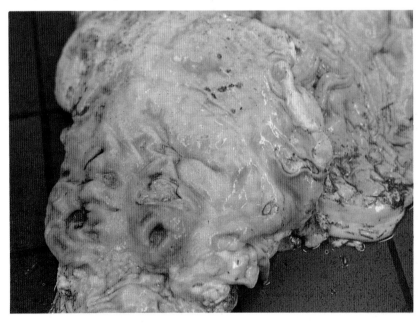

Plate 176 Abomasal Lymphosarcoma

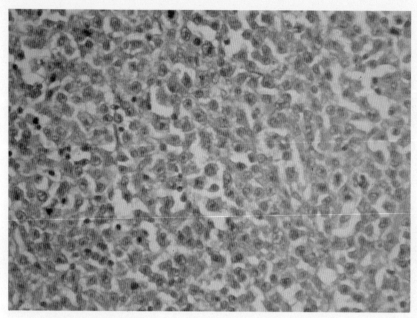

Plate 177   Gastric Lymphosarcoma

A monotonous compact population of large neoplastic lymphocytes has diffusely replaced various structures of the host tissue. Necrotic nuclei are prominent and mitotic figures are frequent. H&E stain.

IX.   Miscellaneous
Cantharidin Toxicosis in Horses

"Blister" beetles belonging to the genus Epicauta when consumed with alfalfa hay frequently are fatal in horses. The beetles contain cantharidin which causes acantholysis and vesicle formation when in contact with skin or mucous membranes. As little as 4 to 6 mg of dead dried Epicauta beetles may kill a horse due most likely to marked hypocalcemia and hypomagnesemia or due to cardiac failure from necrosis of myocardial tissue. The dead beetles become entrapped in alfalfa hay during harvest.   Clinical signs include colic.depression, micturition, hematuria and oral ulceration.   Cantharidin is clinically detected in stomach contents and in urine by gas chromatography or mass spectrometry.   Detection of blister beetles in the hay or of beetle parts in the gastrointestinal contents provides additional diagnostic certainty.

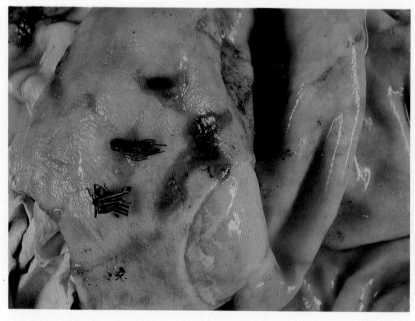

Plates 178-181   Cantharidin Toxicosis

Within the gastrointestinal tract and urothelium, cantharidin causes mucosal vesicles, hemorrhage, erosions and necrosis. Digested insect segments may be detected when present in large numbers.

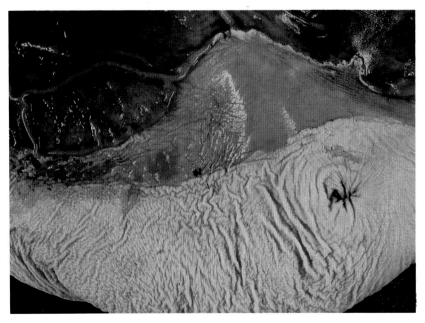

Plate 179 Cantharidin Toxico-sis

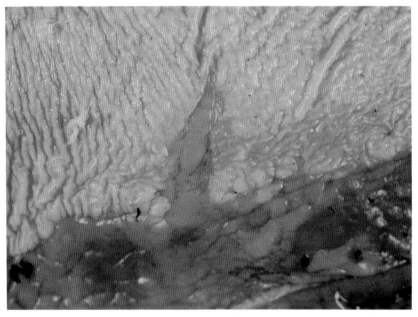

Plate 180 Cantharidin Toxico-sis

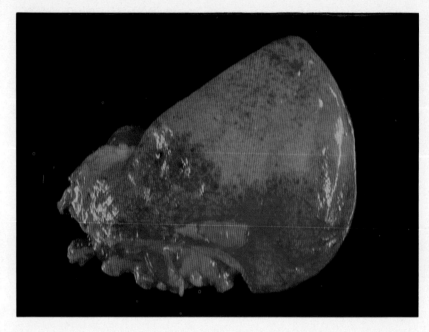

Plate 181 Cantharidin Toxicosis

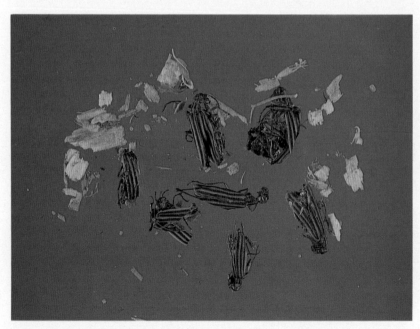

Plate 182 Epicauta Beetle

The majority of blister beetles fatal to horses involve the three-striped blister beetle found in the Southwestern United States.

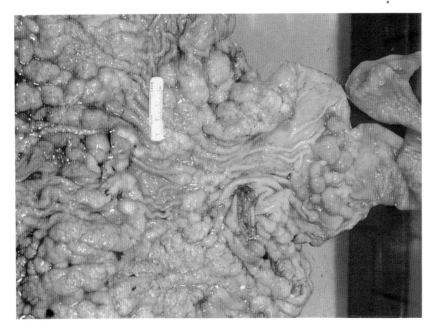

Plates 183,184 Hypertrophic Gastritis

A proliferative gastritis with marked diffuse rugal hypertrophy or solitary antral hypertrophy has been described in the Basenji and other dogs. Clinical findings are weight loss, diarrhea, anemia, hypoproteinemia and hypergammaglobulinemia. The disease resembles Menetrier's disease in man,also known as giant hypertrophic gastritis. The lesions should not be confused with neoplasia of the stomach such as malignant lymphoma or pythiosis. The lesions consist of rugal thickening mimicking the cerebral convolutions.

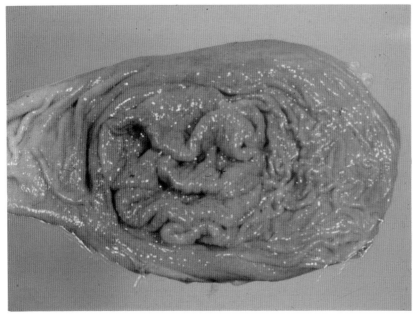

Plate 184 Hypertrophic Gastritis

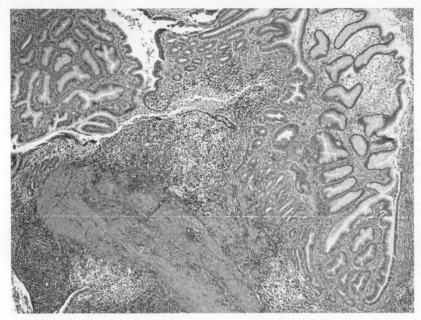

Plates 185, 186   Hypertrophic Gastritis

Microscopically, the affected gastric mucosa is excessively folded due to hyperplasia and occasionally metaplasia. The lamina propria contains lymphocytes and plasma cells mainly, but also neutrophils and eosinophils. H&E stain.

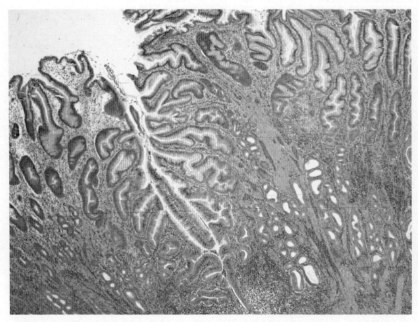

Plate 186 Hypertrophic Gastritis

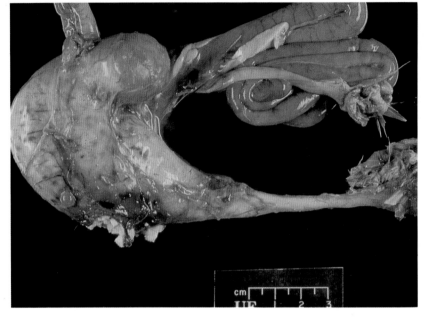

Plate 187 Psittacine Proventricular Dilatation Syndrome

The syndrome was described in the early 1980s and is also known as macaw wasting syndrome since it is most commonly seen in macaws. It can affect other psittacine birds including parrots and cockatoos. Case fatality is nearly 100%.

At necropsy the proventriculus and the duodenum are markedly distended and contain large amounts of impacted indigested food.

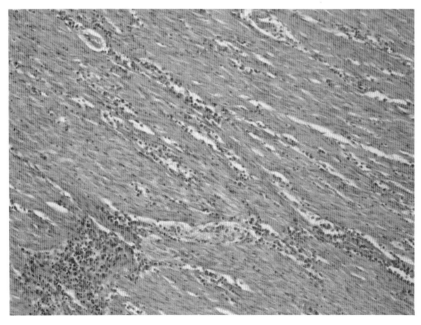

Plates 188,189 Psittacine Proventricular Dilatation Syndrome

Microscopically, mild to moderate lymphoplasmacytic infiltrates are associated with intramural myenteric ganglia. Myenteric ganglionic cells are destroyed. Occasionally, eosinophilic intranuclear and cytoplasmic inclusions are detected suggesting a viral origin. Ultrastructural examination of the inclusions indicated the presence of paramyxovirus.

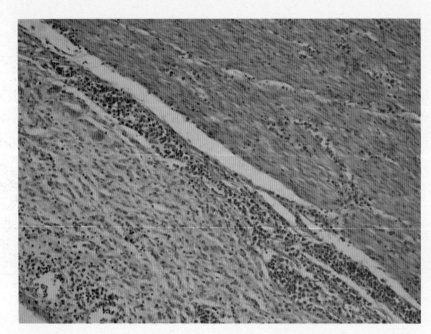

Plate 189 Psittacine Proventricular Dilatation Syndrome

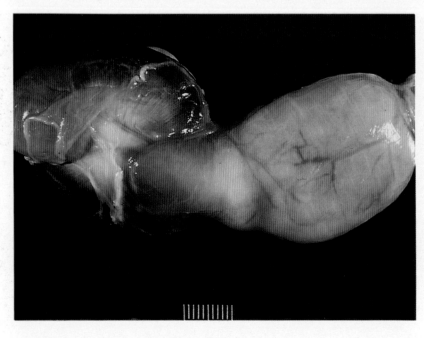

Plate 190 Marek's Disease
In a chicken proventricular thickening and distention commonly result from neoplastic lymphoid infiltrates.

Literature

1 . B.L. Blagburn, D.S. Lindsay, Ch. M. Hendrix, J. Schumacher: Pathogenesis, Treatment and Control of Gastric Parasites in Horses. Comp. Cont. Ed. 13:850, 1991.

2 . C.F. Burrows, L.A. Ignaszewski: Canine Gastric Dilatation -Volvulus. J. Sm. An. Pract. 31:495, 1990.

3 . C.G. Couto, H.C. Rutgers, R.G. Sherding, J. Rojko: Gastrointestinal Lymphoma in 20 Dogs, J. Vet. Int. Med. 3:73, 1989.

4 . M.L. Kiper, J. Traub-Dargatz, Ch. R. Curtis: Gastric Rupture in Horses: 50 Cases (1979-1987). J. Am. Vet. Med. Assoc. 196:333, 1990.

5 . C.L. Meschter, M. Gilbert, L. Krook, G. Maylin, R. Carradino: The Effects of Phenylbutazone on the Intestinal Mucosa of the Horse: A Morphological, Ultrastructural and Biochemical Study. Eq. Vet. J. 22: 255, 1990.

6 . C.L. Meschter, M. Gilbert, L. Krook, G. Maylin, R. Carradino: The Effects of Phenylbutazone on the Morphology and Prostaglandin Concentration of the Pyloric Mucosa of the Equine Stomach. Vet. Path. 27:244, 1990.

7 . N.J. MacLachlan, E.B. Breitschwerdt, J.M. Uanbers, R.E. Agenzio, E.V. DeBuysscher: Gastroenteritis in Basenji Dogs. Vet. Path. 25:36, 1988.

8 . A. Mannl, H. Gerlach, R. Leipold: Neuropathic Gastric Dilatation in Psittaciformes. Av. Dis. 31:214, 1987.

9 . S. Metliyapu, J. Pohlenz, H. Ch. Bertschinger: Ultrastructure of the Intestinal Mucosa in Pigs Experimentally Inoculated With a Edema- Disease Producing Strain of E. coli (0139:K12:H1). Vet. Path. 21:516, 1984.

10. K.J. Moreland: Ulcer Disease of the Upper Gastrointestinal Tract in Small Animals: Pathophysiology, Diagnosis, and Management. Comp. Cont. Ed.10:1265, 1988.

11. M.J. Murray: Endoscopic Appearance of Gastric Lesions in Foals: 94 Cases (1987-1988). J. Am. Vet. Med. Assoc. 195:1135, 1989.

12. M.J. Murray: The Pathogenesis and Prevalence of Gastric Ulceration in Foals and Horses. Vet. Med. 86: 815, 1991.

13. G. Nappert, A. Vrins, M. Larybyere: Gastroduodenal Ulceration in Foals. Comp. Cont. Ed. 11:335, 1989.

14. A. Patnaik: Canine Gastrointestinal Neoplasms. Vet. Path. 14:547, 1977.

15. A. Patnaik: Canine Gastric Adenocarcinomas. Vet. Path. 15:600, 1978.

16. D.G. Schmitz: Cantharidin Toxicosis in Horses. J. Vet. Int. Med. 3:208, 1989.

17. T.R. Schoeb, R.J. Panciera: Pathology of Blister Beetle (Epicauta) Poisoning in Horses. Vet. Path. 16:18, 1979.

Chapter 4 Intestinal Tract

Nutrients and water only become part of the body after they have crossed the lining of the gut and have entered the bloodstream. Thus, structural conditions of the intestinal tract are inseparable from those of function.

I. Structure

The wall of the intestine is composed of four major layers: the mucosa, submucosa, muscularis and serosa. The mucosa is composed of an epithelial layer with a basement membrane, a lamina propria containing blood vessels, lymphatics, smooth muscle cells, nerve fibers and resident cells of the gut-associated immune system. The submucosa contains large blood vessels, lymphatics, connective tissue, nerves, ganglia and lymphatic elements. The muscularis is divided into an inner circular layer and an outer longitudinal layer of smooth muscle cells. The myenteric plexus is interspersed between the two. The serosa is the most outer layer. The mucosa is the most important stratum for the digestion and absorption of nutrients. The small intestine is morphologically differentiated from the large intestine by the presence of villi which project into the intestinal lumen from folds. Between the villi are depressions defined as crypts. Each villus is covered by an epithelium one cell layer thick. Two main cell types make up the villus epithelium: the enterocyte responsible for digestion and absorption and the goblet cell secreting mucus for the protection of the intestinal tract. Cells of both types are produced by cell division in the crypt and migrate to the tip of the villus to resume function.

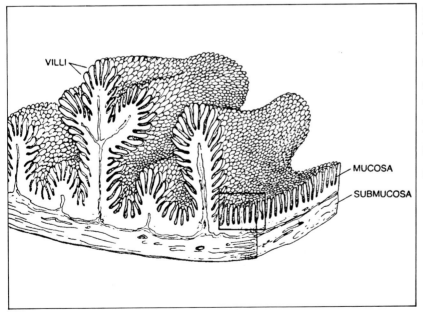

VILLI

MUCOSA

SUBMUCOSA

Plate 191   Intestinal Villi

The foldings of the mucosal surface in conjunction with mucosal villi largely increase the absorptive surface. (From "The Lining of the Small Intestine", by Florence Moog. Copyright (c) 1981 by Scientific American, Inc. All rights reserved.)

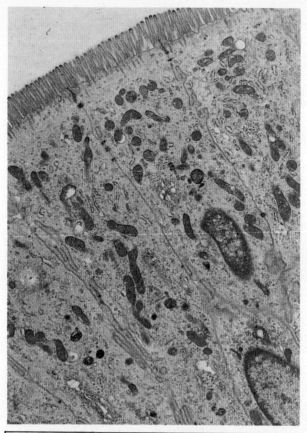

Plate 192   Ultrastructure of Normal Intestinal Epithelium

The low power electron micrograph from normal calf small intestine illustrates the main cell type of the villus:the absorptive enterocyte.

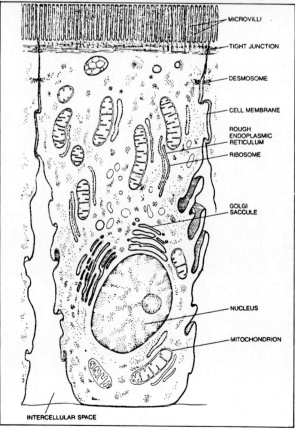

MICROVILLI

TIGHT JUNCTION

DESMOSOME

CELL MEMBRANE

ROUGH ENDOPLASMIC RETICULUM

RIBOSOME

GOLGI SACCULE

NUCLEUS

MITOCHONDRION

INTERCELLULAR SPACE

Plate 193   Schematic Drawing of Enterocyte

Diversified subcellular cytoplasmic organelles facilitate various metabolic functions of enterocytes.   The brush border is a prominent structure on the apical surface of the cell and is made up of microvilli.   (From "The Lining of the Small Intestine", by Florence Moog. Copyright (c) 1981 by Scientific American, Inc.   All rights reserved.)

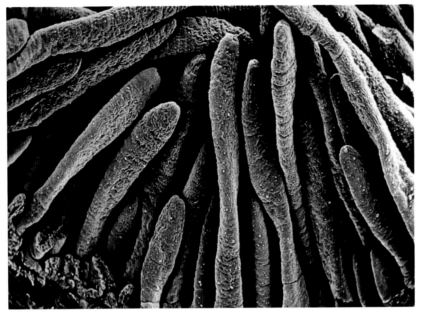

Plate 194   Ultrastructure of Intestinal Villi

The scanning electron micrograph from normal pig jejunal epithelium illustrates villus projections into the intestinal lumen giving the tissue a velvet appearance.

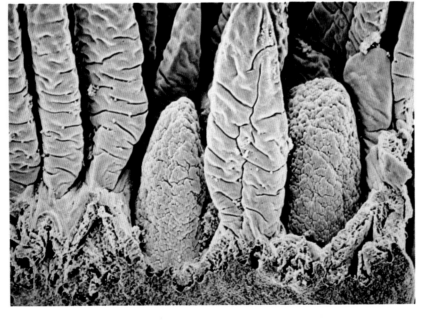

Plate 195   Ultrastructure of Intestinal Villi

The scanning electron micrograph from a normal calf jejunum illustrates villi resting over a Peyer's patch.

II. Function

Digestion and protection from toxins and infectious agents are two of the major functions of the gut. Secretion, digestion, absorption and propulsion are non-immunologic functions. Most absorption and secretion occur in the small intestine. The principal function of the large intestine is absorption of sodium and chloride as well as water, and secretion of mucus.

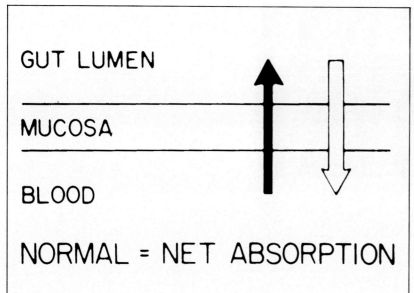

Plate 196   Fluid Flux in Normal Intestinal Mucosa

There are continuous bidirectional fluxes of water and electrolytes across the intestinal mucosa. Secretory fluxes (movement from blood to gut), as well as absorptive fluxes (movement from gut to blood), occur simultaneously. When the entire intestinal tract in a clinically normal animal is considered, absorptive fluxes exceed secretory fluxes, resulting in net absorption. (Reproduced by permission of the Journal of the American Veterinary Medical Association.)

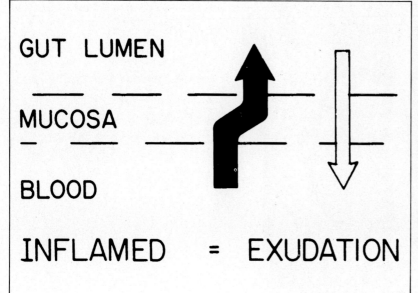

Plate 197   Fluid Flux in Diseased Intestinal Mucosa

Inflammation of the intestine can be accompanied by increased hydraulic pressure and increased flow through the membranes (leak) down the pressure gradient from blood to the intestinal lumen. If the amount of material secreted exceeds the absorptive capacity of the intestine, diarrhea results. (Reproduced by permission of the Journal of the American Veterinary Medical Association.)

Gut-associated Lymphoid Tissue (GALT)

Both cellular and humeral components represent important immunological defense mechanisms in the intestinal tract for protection from pathologic organisms and toxic agents. The tissue from which these elements are derived is known as Peyer's patch.

Peyer's patches are composed of groups of lymphoid follicles which are located below the mucosal epithelium. The density of Peyer's patches is greatest in the ileum. Peyer's patches contain lymphocytes of both B-cell and T-cell lineage. In addition, solitary lymphoid follicles are randomly spread throughout the intestinal mucosa.

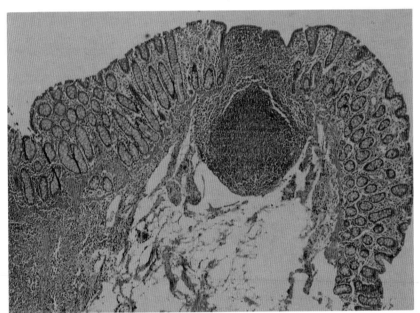

Plate 198 Solitary Lymphoid Follicle

A nodule of aggregated lymphocytes is discretely located in the lamina propria of porcine large intestine.

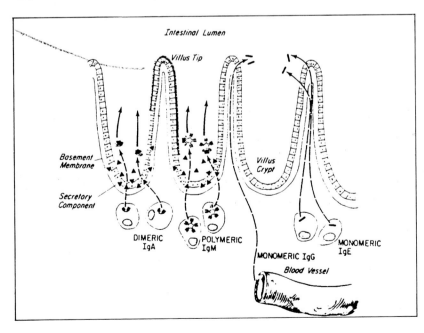

Plate 199 Intestinal Antibodies

Intestinal resident plasma cells are responsible for the production of all classes of immunoglobulins into the intestinal secretion. By far the predominant protective immunoglobulin is IgA which is present in dimeric form. Together with IgM, polymeric immunoglobulins are assembled and transported across the basement membrane onto the intestinal surface. Monomeric immunoglobulins are synthesized locally or transported out of the intestinal circulation into the intestinal lumen. (Reprinted, by permission of the New England Journal of Medicine, Vol. 297, page 768, 1977.)

110

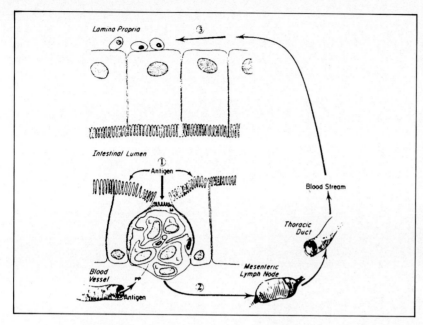

Plate 200 Trafficking of Intestinal T-cells

Intestinal antigens stimulate T-cells associated with GALT. Such stimulated lymphoid cells reach the mesenteric lymph nodes and the systemic circulation to redistribute along the intestinal mucosa as T-lymphocytes or IgA secreting plasma cells. (Reprinted. by permission of the New England Journal of Medicine. Vol. 325. page 332. 1991.)

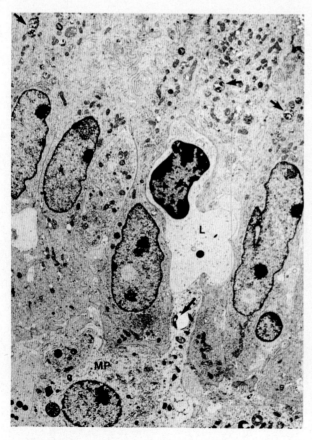

Plate 201 Intestinal M Cells

Membranous epithelial (M) cells or microfold cells are specialized epithelial cells overlying the subepithelial lymphoid follicles of the alimentary tract.Certain bacteria and viruses are known to penetrate the mucosal barrier through M cells with subsequent transport to the Peyer's patches. As part of GALT. the M cell is surrounded by absorptive enterocytes and goblet cells.Morphologically. M cells are characterized by an absence of glycocalyx and by a paucity of microvilli and cytoplasmic organelles such as lysosomes.The M cell represents an important pathway for the direct transport of intestinal macromolecules and antigens to the gut-associated lymphoid tissue. The electron micrograph represents M cells from the intestinal tract of a calf.Notice the close vicinity to lymphoid (L) cells and macrophages(MP) as well as the separation from adjacent enterocytes by tight junctional complexes (arrow).

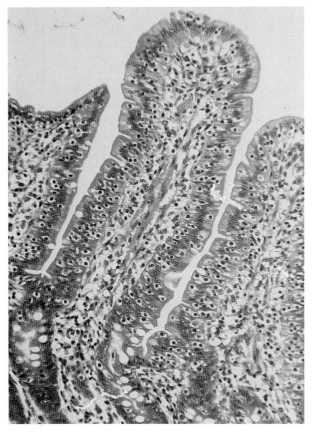

Plate 202   Intraepithelial Lymphocytes

Random distribution of individual lymphocytes in villus epithelium and subepithelium.

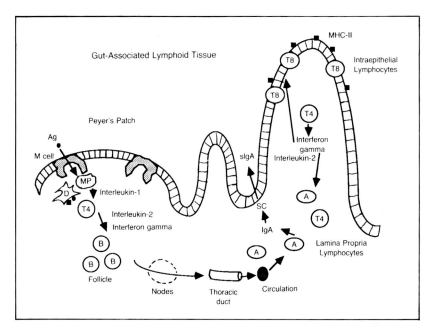

Plate 203   Effector Mechanism in GALT

The diagram represents immunologic events in Peyer's patches starting with the uptake of foreign antigen via special epithelial cells known as microfold (M) cells, the presentation of antigen to subepithelial macrophages and dendritic cells and the processing of antigen by helper (T4) lymphocytes. The production of cytokines affects the maturation of plasma cells and special intraepithelial lymphocytes of defined lineage. The GALT, absorptive enterocyte and goblet cells constitute the mucosal barrier system.

III. Intestinal Anomalies

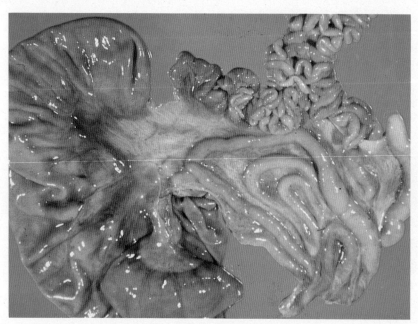

Plate 204   Jejunal Atresia

Aplasia, hypoplasia and atresia occur in various segments of the intestine, but preferentially affect colon, rectum and anus. The arrow identifies the blindly ending segments in the jejunum of a calf with accumulation of ingesta in the cranial portion. The condition in calves has been reported to be due to vascular insufficiency in the developing fetal gut and can be induced by rectal palpation of the conceptus during early pregnancy of cows.

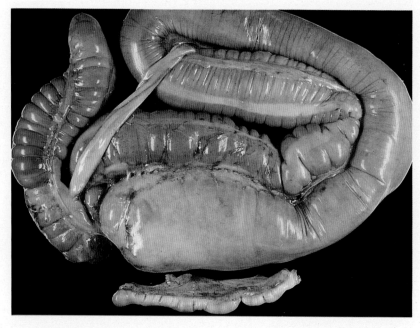

Plate 205 Atresia Coli

Notice a distended large colon in this foal and a very narrow small colon.

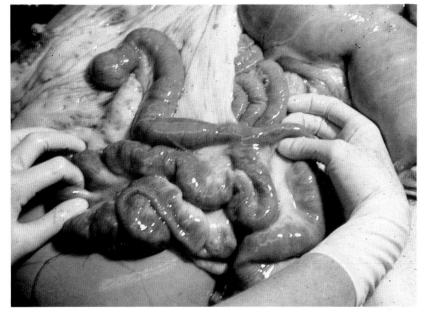

Plate 206   Meckel's Diverticulum

It is defined as vestigial remnant of the proximal omphalomesenteric (vitelline) duct and is found to be attached as a tube-like structure to the ileum of horses, swine and sheep as shown here. In swine and sheep it may be up to 30 cm in length. Its mucosal lining is similar to that of the ileum.

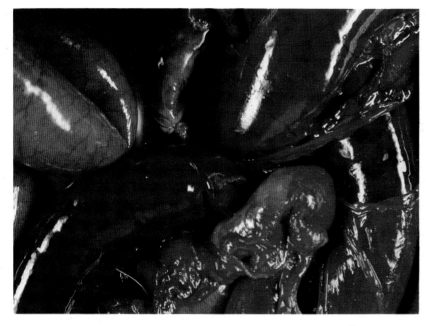

Plate 207   Meckel's Diverticulum

Though usually diagnosed as an incidental finding, it can occasionally give rise to intestinal strangulation as happened to this horse

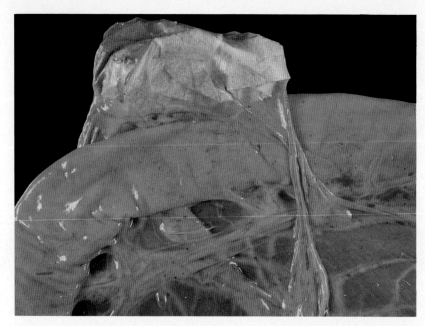

Plate 208 Mesodiverticular Band

A fibrous band drapes around the jejunum of a horse from one side of the mesentery to the other. The mesodiverticular band is thought to be the vestigial remnant of vitelline vessels.

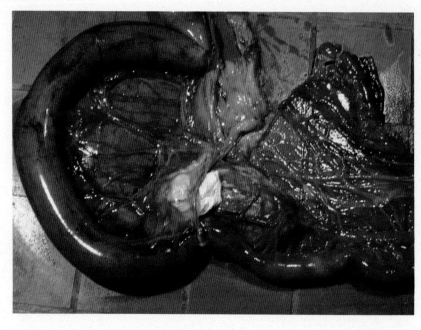

Plate 209 Mesodiverticular Band

This horse suffered from severe incarceration of the small intestine due to ligation by a thin band.

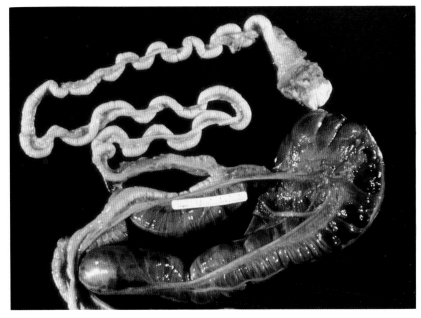

Plates 210,211 Equine Ileocolonic Aganglionosis

The absence of myenteric ganglia in the terminal ileum, cecum and entire colon in white foals born to overo spotted parents is known as "Lethal White Foal" syndrome. The syndrome is associated with colic and death shortly after birth. The almost white foal is of overo color pattern. Its colon is markedly impacted due to meconium retention.

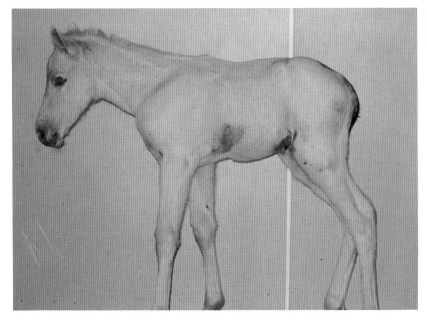

Plate 211 Equine Ileocolonic Aganglionosis

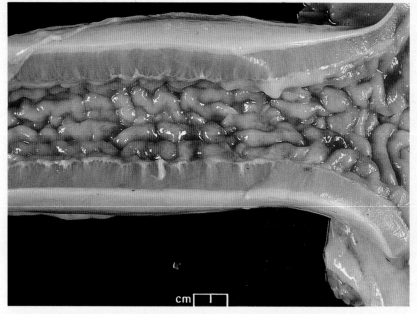

Plates 212,213 Ileal Hypertrophy

The condition occurs as muscular hypertrophy in swine and horses and as mucosal hypertrophy in sheep. It is uncertain whether it is congenital or acquired, and it has been hypothesized that the muscular form of hypertrophy is secondary to, possibly neurogenic, stenosis of the ileocecal valve. The close-up view of ileal muscular hypertrophy is from a horse. It shows the mucosa thrown into thick, encephaloid folds. On cut-section it becomes evident that the thickness of the ileal wall is due to a prominent tunica muscularis.

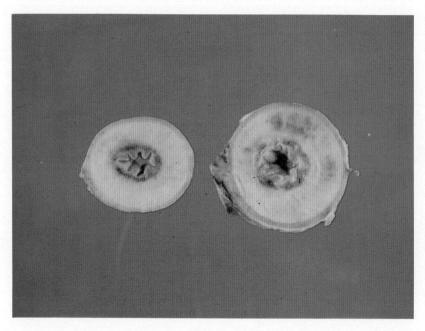

Plate 213 Ileal Hypertrophy

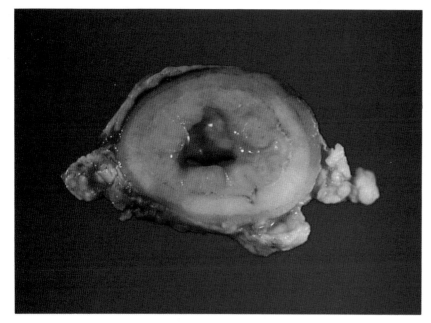

Plates 214,215   Ileal Hypertrophy

Sporadic case of muscular thickening in a sow. Normal porcine ileum is added for comparison.

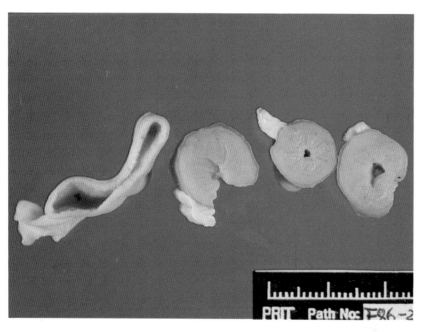

Plate 215   Ileal Hypertrophy

IV. Intestinal Obstruction

The higher (more cranial) the obstruction within the intestinal tract, the more acute are the clinical signs and the more rapid is the clinical course.The latter is associated with loss of water and electrolytes and with venous stasis. Cardiovascular collapse frequently is the cause of death. The vast majority of intestinal obstruction is the result of mechanical disturbances;of lesser frequency are vascular or neurogenic causes. Examples of mechanical disorders are illustrated in Plates 216 - 245.

(a) mechanical

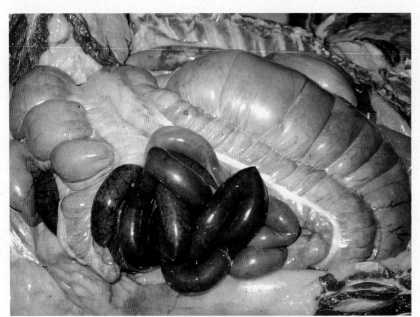

Plates 216,217 Volvulus

Rotations around the mesenteric attachment develops with significant frequency in species with a long intestinal tract such as the horse. Death occurs frequently if therapeutic intervention is delayed. The affected intestinal loops are of dark, red-blue color due to venous engorgement and obstruction. Gangrene of the intestinal wall is the result of vascular flow interference.

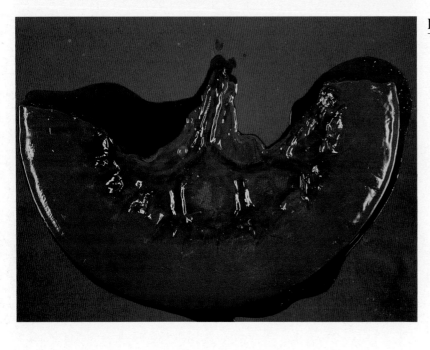

Plate 217 Volvulus

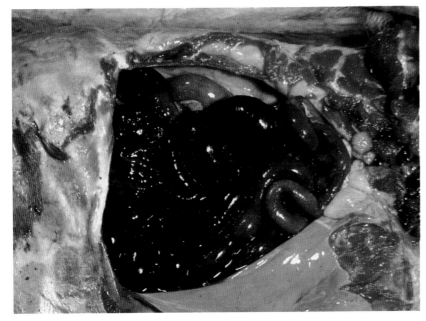

Plate 218　Volvulus

Large-breed dogs are also prone to the development of intestinal twists.

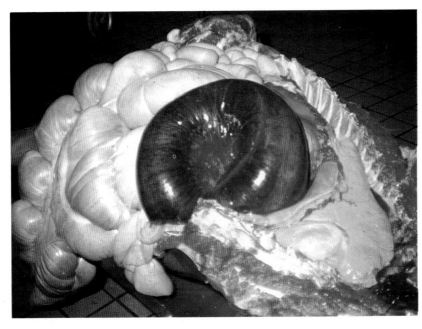

Plates 219,220　Torsion

The large colon has rotated around its longitudinal axis in this horse.As with volvulus there is severe devitalization of tissue. The colonic wall is thickened and will pit with pressure. Most equine torsions are clockwise and can be up to 540 degree. The free loops of the ventral left and right large colon segments are clearly demarcated from the more fixed dorsal loops which did not rotate. In the cow. cecal torsion can be encountered.

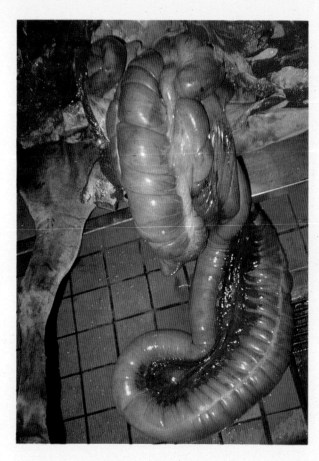

Plate 220 Torsion

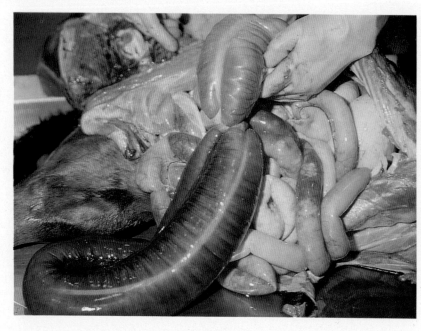

Plate 221 Torsion
Colonic torsion in a foal.

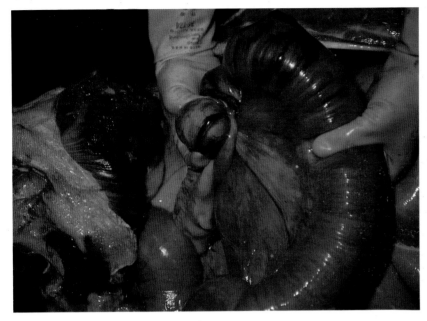

Plates 222–225 Strangulating Lipoma

Lipomas arise from the serosal or mesenteric surfaces usually of obese, older horses. As they grow, lipomas change from a sessile to a pedunculated form to wrap around the intestinal tube causing strangulation. Larger lipomas may outgrow their blood supply by twisting around the peduncle and to undergo ischemic necrosis changing color and composition.

Plate 223 Strangulating Lipoma

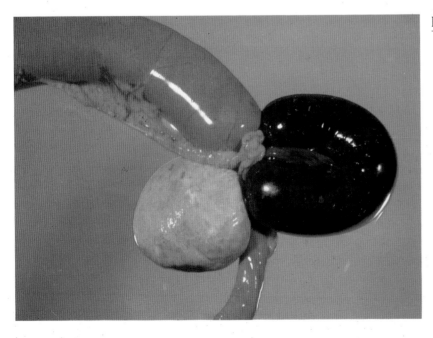

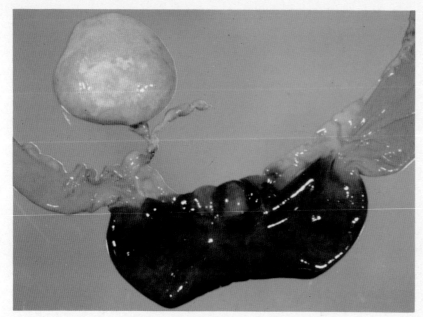

Plate 224   Strangulating Lipoma

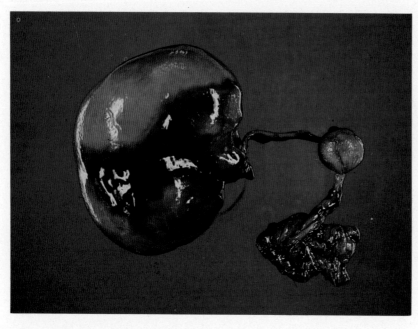

Plate 225   Strangulating Lipoma

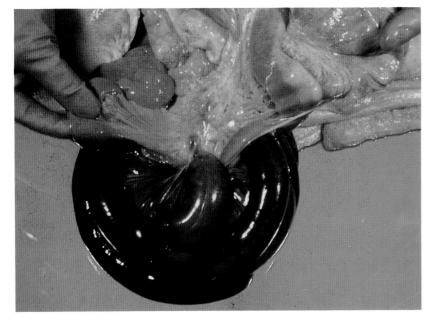

Plates 226–228 Intestinal "Knotting"

Portions of the jejunal loops have knotted around themselves in this pig. probably due to a rent in the mesentery.

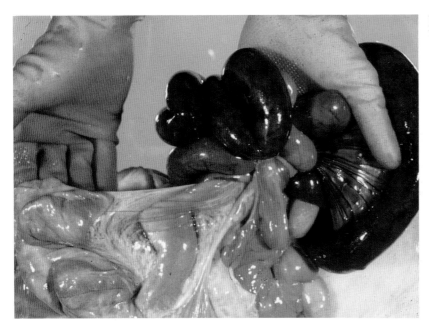

Plate 227   Intestinal "Knotting"

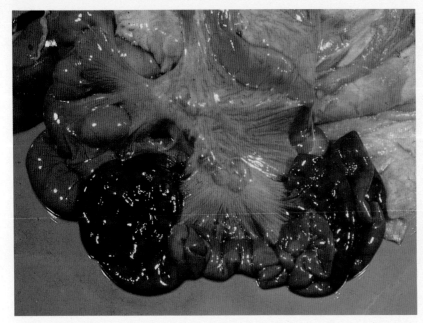

Plate 228   Intestinal "Knotting"

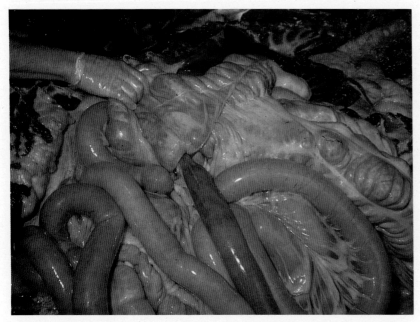

Plate 229   Intussusception

Intussusception is defined as telescoping of one section of intestine into an other. It occurs commonly in dogs, cattle and sheep and is often, but not necessarily, associated with enteritis or endoparasitism. This is ileal intussusception near the ileocecal junction in a foal. Vascular compromise is indicated by serosal reddening.

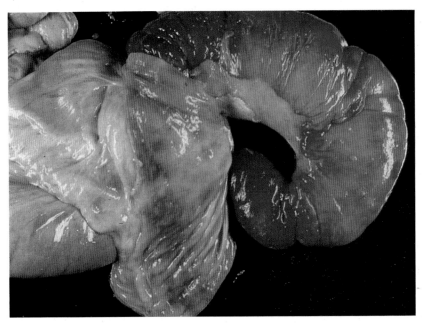

Plate 230 Intussusception

Cecocolonic telescoping in a calf as the result of peri-intestinal abscessation. The contained intestinal segment swells and becomes adherent; soon it becomes necrotic and gangrenous. The recipient segment in intussusception is called the intussuscipiens; the telescoping segment is called intussusceptum. Most unattended intestinal invaginations are fatal.

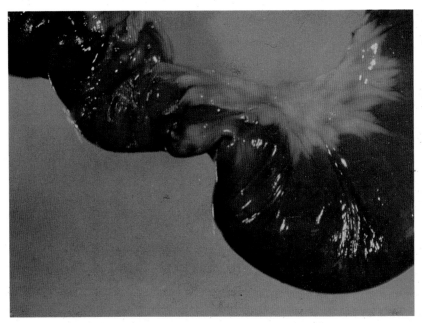

Plate 231 Intussusception

Jejunal intussusception in a sheep secondary to heavy infestation with Oesophagostomum sp.

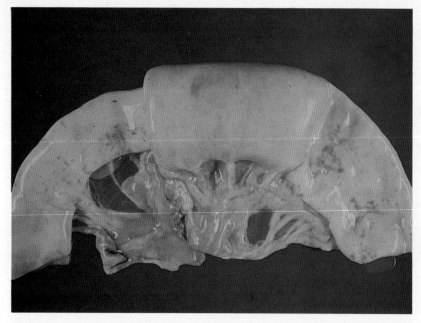

Plate 232 Postmortem Invagination

After death intestinal segments may telescope. The invaginating segments lack tissue adhesion or vascular compromise unlike antemortem intussusception.

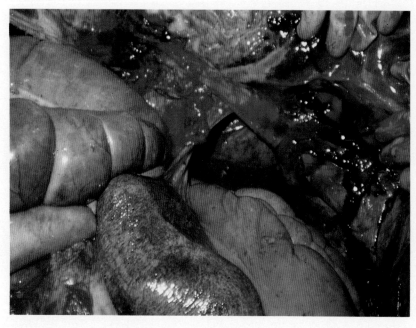

Plate 233 Nephrosplenic Ligament

In this horse portions of the small intestine became entrapped and strangulated in a fold between the spleen and the left kidney.

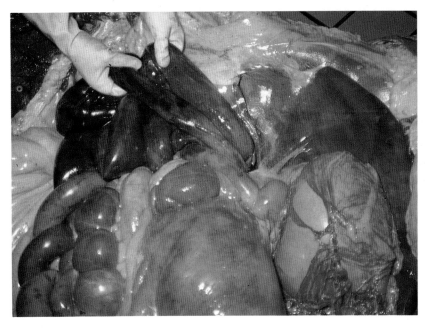

Plate 234 Foramen Epiploicum

Portions of equine small intestine have slipped into a loose gap between the caudal liver, duodenum and stomach. Strangulation is the result.

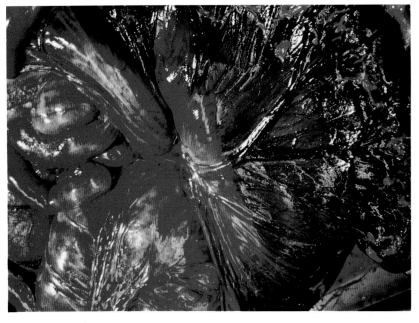

Plate 235 Mesenteric Rents

Tears in the mesentery facilitate intestinal strangulation as in this horse.

Intraluminal Foreign Bodies

Intestinal foreign bodies not only are the cause for obstruction but also may be responsible for perforations and ruptures leading to fatal peritonitis.

Examples of intestinal foreign bodies are:

    Sand impaction
    Sharp objects
    Blunt objects
    Concrements, e.g. enteroliths, fecaliths
    Phyto- or trichobezoars

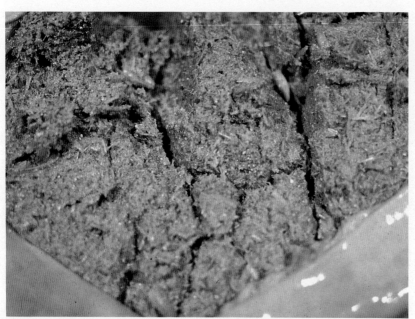

Plates 236,237 Sand Impaction

Sand enteropathy in horses occurs when animals are kept on pasture rich in sand instead of grass. Sand has a tendency to settle in the large colon and cecum making the organ very heavy. A large volume of sand may overwhelm the ability of the tract to clear itself. As it accumulates, sand causes irritation of the entire intestinal wall ultimately causing rupture and peritonitis.

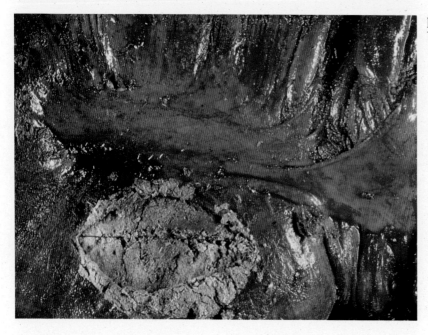

Plate 237   Sand Impaction

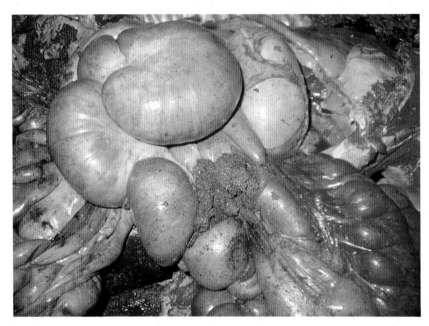

Plate 238   Cecal Rupture

An impacted cecum is the second most frequent site of the gastrointestinal tract to rupture and a cause of sudden death in the horse. The cecum typically ruptures at the base on either the medial or lateral side.

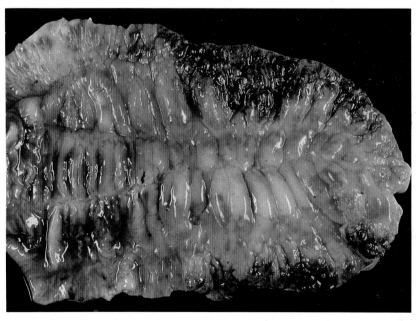

Plate 239   Meconium Impaction

Meconium usually is evacuated by the newborn foal in the first few hours after parturition. Meconium retention is clinically recognized by restlessness and the inability to defecate. Such retained meconium may irritate the mucosa.

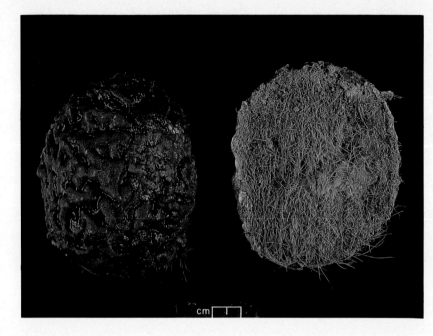

Plates 240,241 Phytobezoar

These are examples of dried fecaliths of plant origin as they may become entrapped in the large intestinal tract without leading to clinical complications.

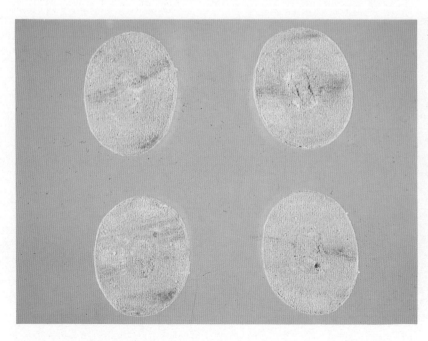

Plate 241   Phytobezoar

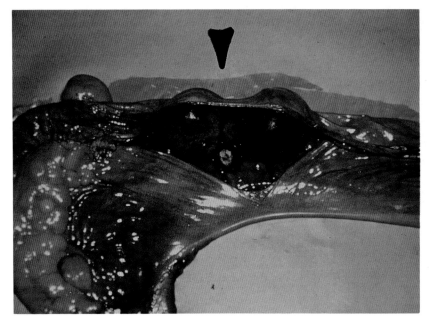

Plates 242,243   Enteroliths

Mineral enteroliths (arrow) in the right dorsal colon of a horse. The development of an enterolith depends on the presence of salts, a nidus for precipitation and some degree of intestinal sluggishness. Enteroliths may become very heavy and large and may be the cause of obstruction and perforation when they cannot be passed through intestinal narrowings such as the transition into the transverse colon or the pelvic flexure.

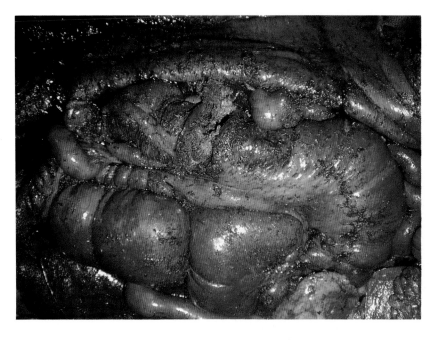

Plate 243   Enteroliths

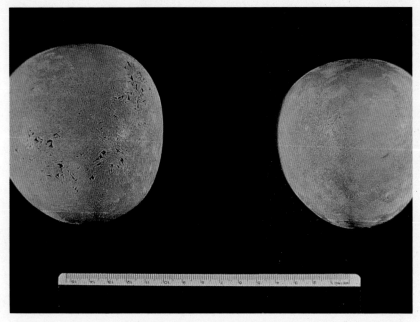

Plates 244,245　Enteroliths

Intestinal calculi usually are composed of ammonium magnesium phosphate. The source of the magnesium phosphate is grain containing large amounts of salts. In chronic gastrointestinal diseases. large amounts of unsplit salt escape to the colon to combine with ammonia.produced as the result of bacterial digestion of protein. to form ammonium magnesium phosphate. On cut-section. enteroliths show the composition of lamellated layers. 1 ～ 2 mm thick.

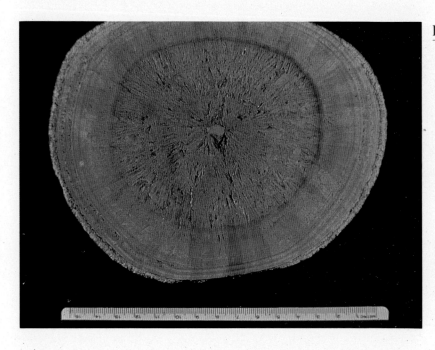

Plate 245　Enteroliths

(b) Vascular

Vascular-induced intestinal obstructions are the result of thrombi or emboli in mesenteric vessels. The classical example is verminous arteritis of the cranial mesenteric root causing recurrent colic in the horse.

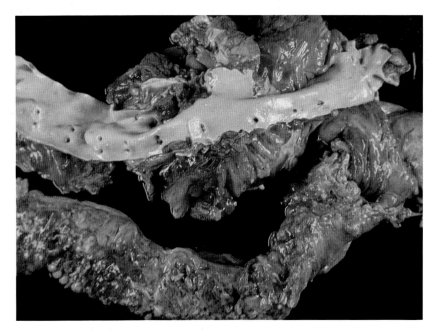

Plate 246 Verminous Arteritis

The severe thrombotic and inflammatory changes in the cranial mesenteric root and within the ileocecocolonic arterial tributary is the result of migrating larvae of Strongylus vulgaris. The abdominal aorta is uninvolved.

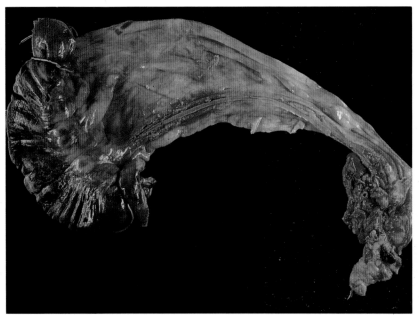

Plates 247,248 Recurrent Colic

Emboli occluding major portions of the colonic artery are responsible for intestinal infarcts in the pelvic flexure of this horse. Infarcts are greenish or red.

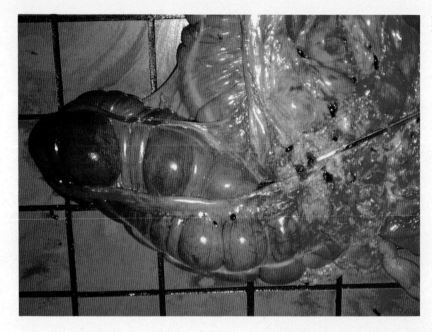

Plate 248   Recurrent Colic

(c) Neurogenic

Neurogenic-induced obstruction may develop after abdominal surgery, trauma or in conjunction with severe peritonitis (paralytic ileus). Grass sickness in the horse is a disease with clinical signs of colic, tympany, salivation and excessive sweating.

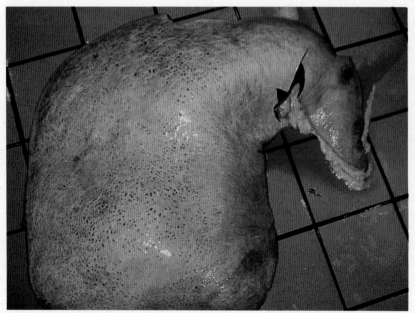

Plate 249   Grass Sickness

Gross findings in grass sickness are fluid-filled stomach, fluid-filled intestine and splenomegaly as illustrated in the Plate. Microscopically, ganglion cell degeneration is present in the splanchnic myenteric ganglia close to the adrenals.

V. Intestinal Dilatation

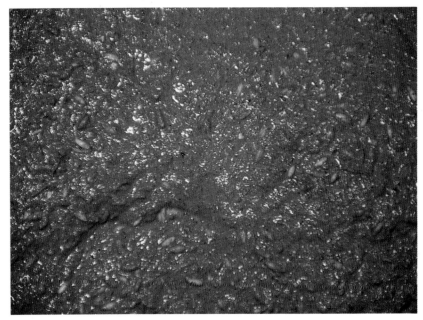

Plate 250 Acute Tympany (Meteorism)

Gas distention of the large colon and cecum is the usual form of alimentary bloating in young horses "pushed" with carbohydrate-rich feed.

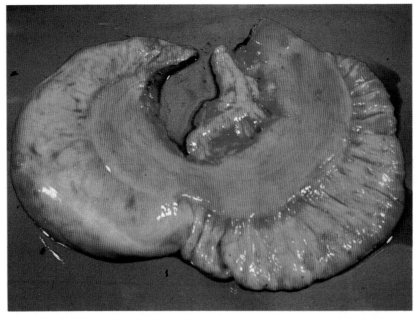

Plates 251,252 Propulsion Diverticulum

Diverticula are herniations of the mucosa into the serosa. The entire intestinal wall thus may consist of little more than mucosa plus serosa. The more diverticula or the longer the diverticulum, the greater the opportunity there is for fecaliths or for inflammation with hemorrhage, obstruction or perforation to develop. True or traction may be distinguished from false or propulsion diverticula. A true diverticulum includes all layers of the gutwall; a false diverticulum involves only herniation of the tunica muscularis. Notice the round, focal outpouching in the ileum of this horse. Subserosal plaques (hemomelasma ilei) are additional findings.

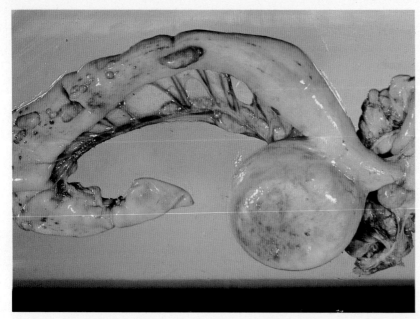

Plate 252 Propulsion Diverticulum

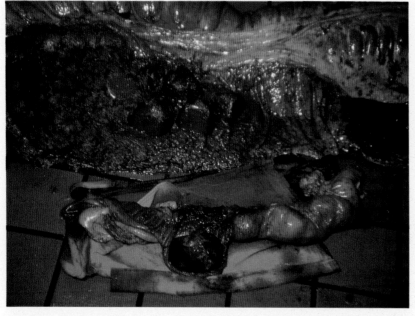

Plate 253   Colonic Enteroliths and Diverticulum

This horse has several enteroliths inside the large colon and an outpouching of the small colon   that includes an entrapped smaller enterolith.

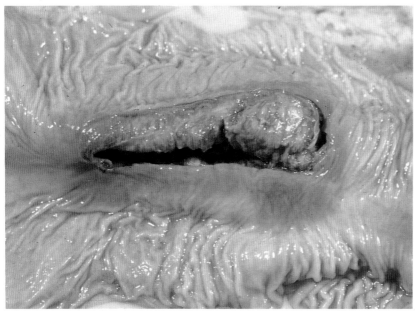

Plate 254 Rectal Perforation

Obstetrical intervention, sadism, or faulty rectal palpation may result in rectal tears of varying degree with rectal perforation being the most severe complication.

VI. Inflammation

Intestinal inflammation can be classified according to:

1. site: duodenitis; proctitis.
2. depth: enteritis superficialis; enteritis profunda.
3. tissue response: catarrhal, mucinous, hemorrhagic, necrotic, fibrinous, purulent, granulomatous, proliferative.
4. time course: acute; chronic
5. etiologic agents: viral; bacterial; parasitic; mycotic; toxic.

Overlaps are frequent and limit clear-cut separations.   Enteric inflammations are most conveniently classified according to morphologic appearance and time course.

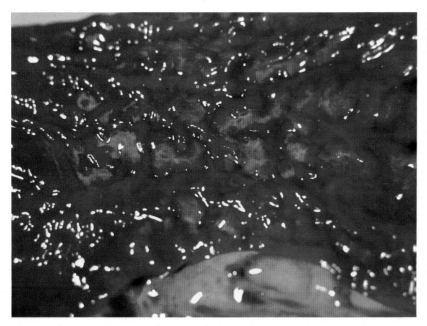

Plate 255 Example of Acute (Exudative) Enteritis in a Horse

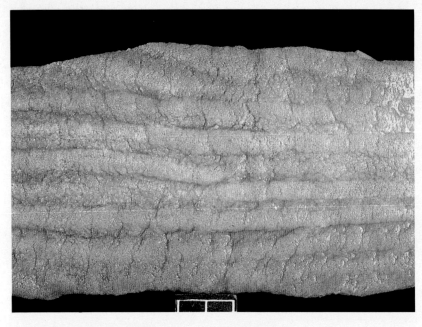

Plate 256   Example of Chronic (Cellular) Enteritis in a Dog

(a)   Secretory (Catarrhal) Enteritis

The cardinal clinical signs of acute secretory enteritis are diarrhea and dehydration.   There are minimal morphologic alterations in the mucosa.   The intestines are flaccid and filled with copious fluid.   The fluid is rich in sodium, chloride and bicarbonates. There is a toxin-induced activation of adenyl cyclase within the brush border of the intestinal epithelial cells with functional impact on cyclic AMP.   The imbalance between secretion and absorption leads to net secretion.   The classic example for secretory enteritis is human cholera caused by Vibrio cholerae.   Certain enteric viral and bacterial animal diseases qualify for this type of enteritis as well.

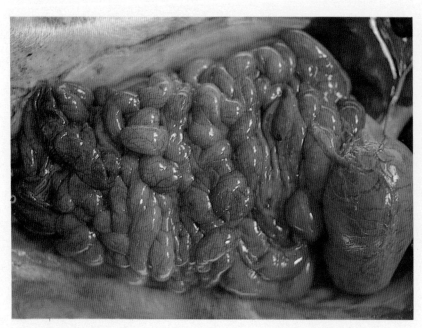

Plate 257 Secretory (Catarrhal) Enteritis in Pig

Morphological signs for acute catarrhal enteritis e.g. inflammation may be extremely difficult to detect, even by microscopic examination.   Catarrhal inflammation is usually more severe at one end of the intestine than at the other.

Viral Enteritis of the Neonate

Rotaviruses and coronaviruses are associated with enteric disease of calves, piglets and foals. The virus attacks the absorptive enterocyte and permits overgrowth by pathogenic bacteria or Cryptosporidium. Gross changes are usually non-specific. Villous atrophy is not much accentuated microscopically.

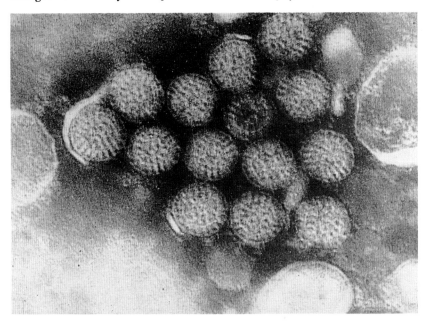

Plate 258   Porcine Rotavirus

The diagnosis is made by demonstrating negatively stained virus particles in feces under the electron microscope.

Transmissible Gastroenteritis of Swine (TGE)

TGE is a frequent cause of death in suckling baby pigs one to two weeks of age. This coronavirus disease is associated with villous atrophy. Cryptal epithelium continues to proliferate. Older pigs are more resistant, but occasionally may become infected with the virus.

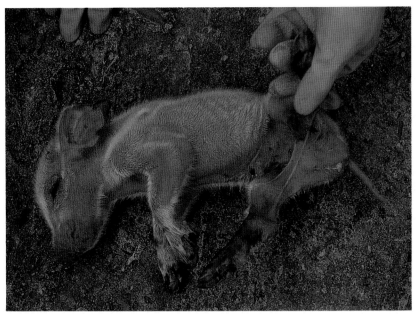

Plate 259   TGE

The slide is from a nine-day-old piglet which died of TGE. Watery feces have stained the entire back portion of the body.

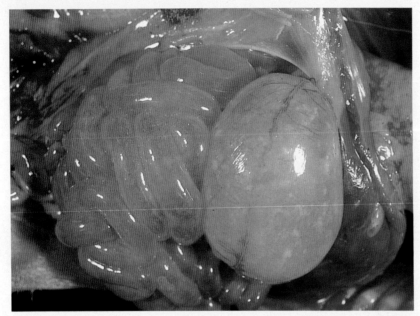

Plate 260   TGE

The small intestinal loops are ballooned and contain flecks of yellow feces. Frequently the intestinal tract is empty while the stomach is filled with food.

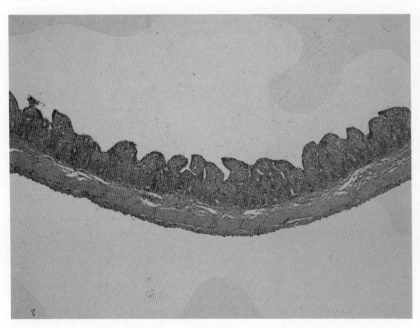

Plates 261,262   TGE

Histologically, TGE is characterized by villous atrophy, blunting and fusion. H&E stain.

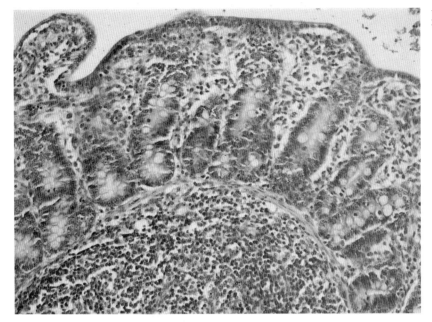

Plate 262   TGE

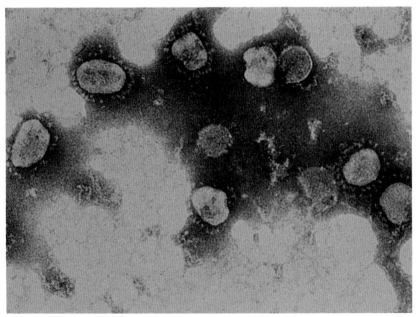

Plate 263   TGE

Electron micrograph of negatively stained coronavirus obtained from feces of piglet with TGE illustrates transmembrane glyco-protein and central nucleoprotein.

142

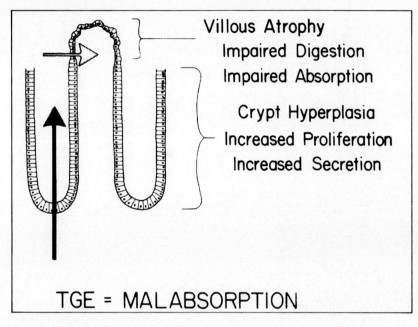

Villous Atrophy
Impaired Digestion
Impaired Absorption

Crypt Hyperplasia
Increased Proliferation
Increased Secretion

TGE = MALABSORPTION

Plate 264   TGE

TGE is associated with malabsorption from reduced villus surface. (Reproduced by permission of the Journal of the American Veterinary Medical Association.)

Colibacillosis

Caused by several serotypes of pathogenic Escherichia coli. Seen in a variety of animal species, notably in neonates. Insufficient colostrum and dietary errors are important precipitating factors.

1. Enterotoxic colibacillosis-enterotoxins accumulate in lumen of small intestine. Strains have ability to adhere to intestinal mucosa by pili. Diagnosis is made by checking for K 99 antigen (adhesin).

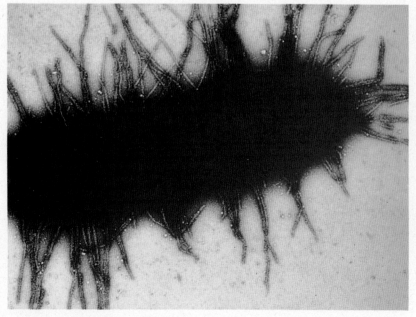

Plate 265   E. coli with Pili

Ultrastructure of adhesive E. coli bacillus.

2. Enterotoxemic colibacillosis-vasotoxins and neurotoxins are produced and absorbed. There is evidence of vascular leakage. Edema disease of weanling swine caused by a hemolytic strain of E. coli belongs to this group.

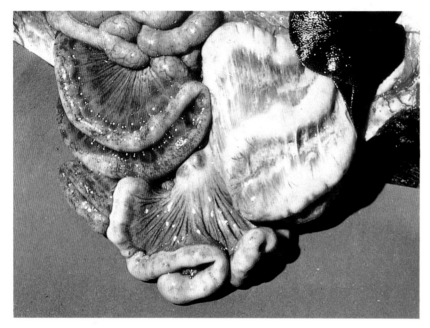

Plates 266-268 Edema Disease
Fibrinoid vascular lesions in several organ systems are responsible for the edema formation. H&E stain.

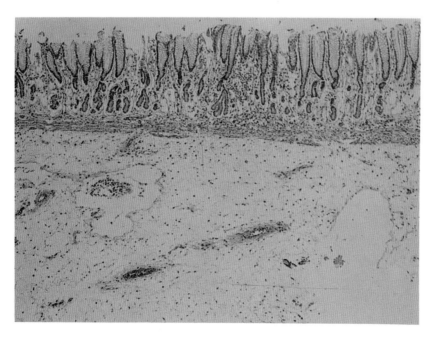

Plate 267 Edema Disease

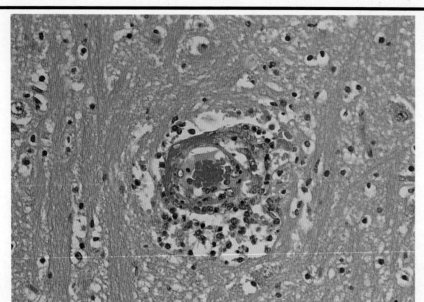

Plate 268   Edema Disease

3. <u>Enteroinvasive</u> <u>colibacillosis</u>-pathogenic agents cause ulceration of the intestinal epithelium through invasion.   There is evidence of fever and dysentery.

4. <u>Systemic</u> <u>colibacillosis</u>-particularly seen in neonatal pigs and calves in antibody deficient state. The mortality rate is almost 100%. The presence of fetid, watery feces is a good indicator for this disorder. It is associated with hypovolemic shock. Hemoconcentration, dehydration, metabolic acidosis are additional clinical findings.   Hyperkalemia causing bradycardia is frequently the cause of death.

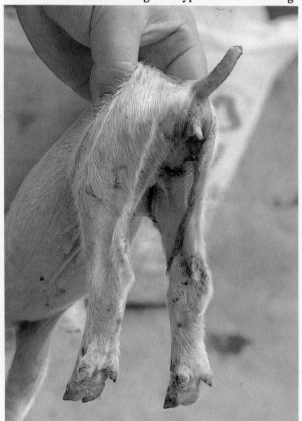

Plate 269   Colibacillosis
Pasting of anus and tail of neonate should suggest the presence of enteric pathogens, but not necessarily <u>E. coli</u>.

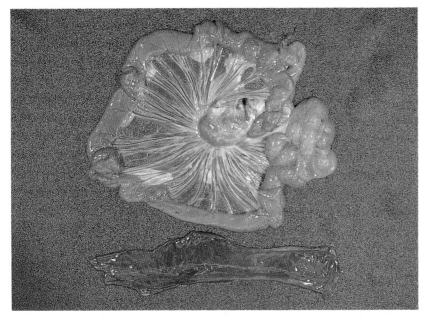

Plate 270   Colibacillosis

The entire small intestinal tract in this piglet is distended by watery feces. The exposed intestinal mucosa is hyperemic.

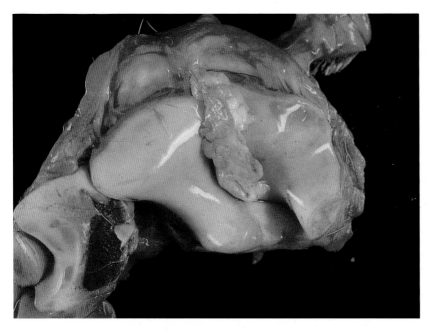

Plate 271   Colibacillosis

Fibrin tags may develop in the hock, stifle and atlanto-occipital joints of calves with diarrhea and are good indicators for the diagnosis of calf septicemia.

146

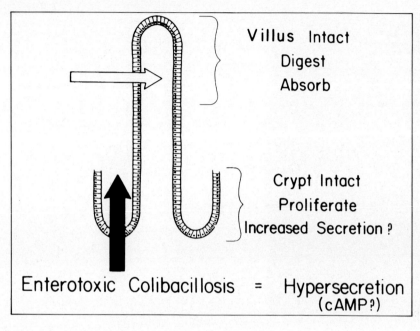

Plate 272 Intestinal Hypersecretion

Schematic drawing to demonstrate pathophysiology of hypersecretion in colibacillosis. (Reproduced by permission of the Journal of the American Veterinary Medical Association.)

(b) Mucinous Enteritis

A good example of this type of inflammation is mucoid enteritis of rabbits. No significant pathologic changes are present at the microscopic level. Only a relative increase in the number of goblet cells has been reported in the ileum. Clinicopathologic findings are leukocytosis, hyperglycemia and electrolyte loss.

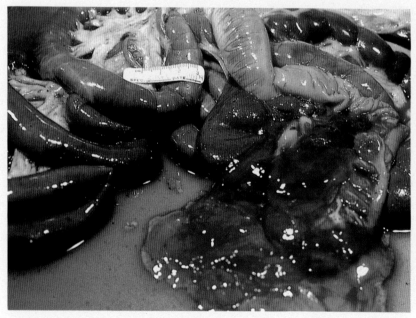

Plates 273,274 Mucoid Enteritis

Grossly, mucus casts are diagnostic of mucoid rabbit enteropathy.

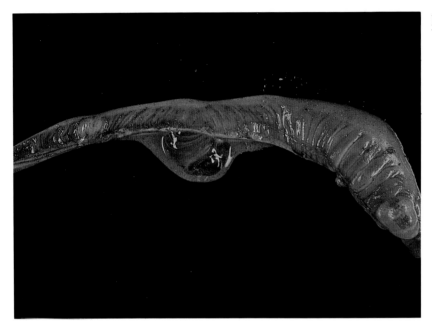

Plate 274   Mucoid Enteritis

(c) Hemorrhaglc Enteritis

The villi are denuded in this type of inflammatory response. The lacteals and superficial capillaries are necrotic and often thrombosed.   There is extravasation of red blood cells into the lamina propria and the lumen of the bowel suggesting vascular permeability disturbance.

Winter Dysentery of Cattle

The sporadic disease is associated with acute diarrhea.transient fever and leukopenia as it typically occurs during the winter season. Adult animals are usually affected.   Coronavirus infection is currently regarded as the most probable cause.   The agent can be demonstrated by electronmicroscopy in feces from affected animals.

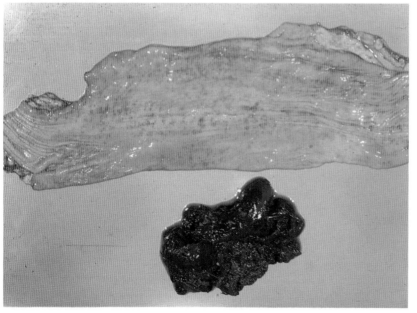

Plate 275   Winter Dysentery

Colon from cow with winter dysentery. Note the absence of significant gross changes except for mild edema and mucosal hemorrhage that occasionally results in intraluminal blood clots.

Clostridial Enterotoxemia

The clostridial enterotoxemias are diseases of young cattle, sheep, goats,horses and pigs and are caused by exotoxins of <u>Clostridium</u> <u>perfringens</u>. Types A-E of exotoxins are distinguished. Types B and C can cause pathologic changes within the intestinal tract. Type D causes diarrhea.

Type B — Causes lamb dysentery. It is also isolated from calves and foals.

Type C — Is isolated from lambs and calves. Responsible for hemorrhagic enteritis of suckling pigs with necrosis of intestinal mucosa.

Type D — Is responsible for "pulpy kidney" disease of lambs. The kidneys are dark and mushy.

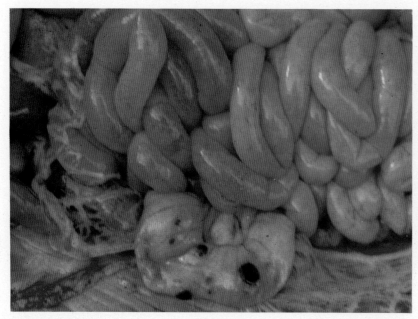

Plates 276,277 Ovine Enterotoxemia

Intestines are distended with gas. Ecchymotic hemorrhages are visible on serosal surfaces.

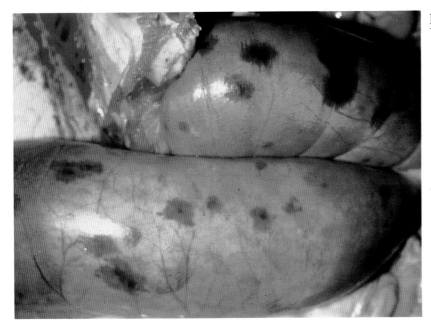

Plate 277 Ovine Enterotoxemia

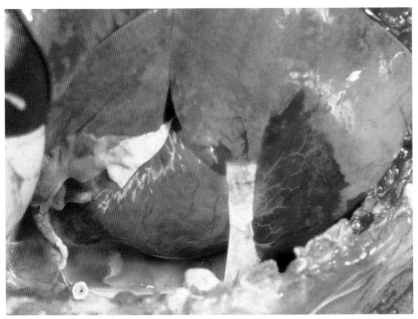

Plate 278 Ovine Enterotoxemia
Fibrinous flakes (arrow) in the pericardial sac are highly indicative of clostridial infection.

150

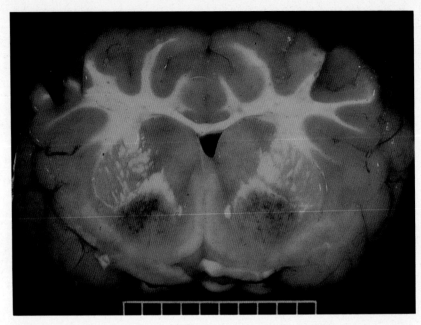

Plate 279   Ovine Enterotoxemia
Bilateral symmetrical foci of hemorrhage and malacia of the thalamus in sheep with enterotoxemia account for convulsions, opisthotonos and coma.

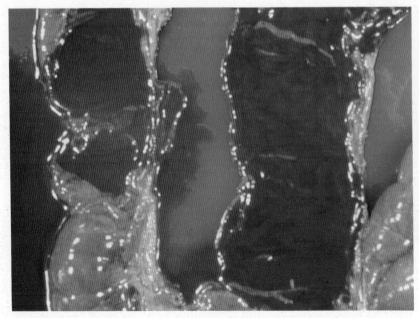

Plates 280,281   Calf Enterotoxemia
The lumen of the small intestine is filled with watery, red fluid. The serosal surfaces are deeply reddened.

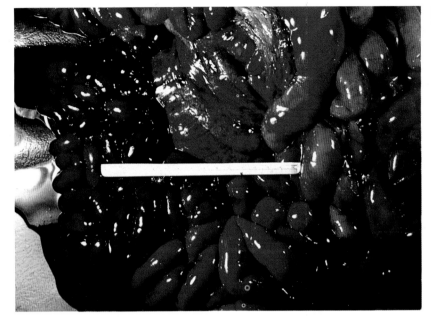

Plate 281   Calf Enterotoxemia

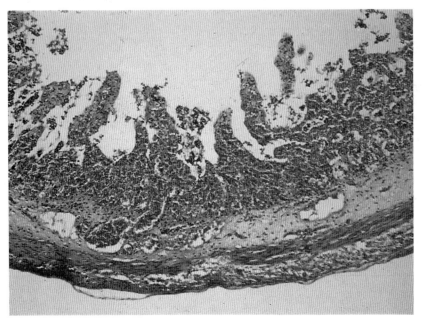

Plate 282   Calf Enterotoxemia

Microscopically, diffuse coagulative necrosis is present in the mucosa. Veins are markedly congested. H&E stain.

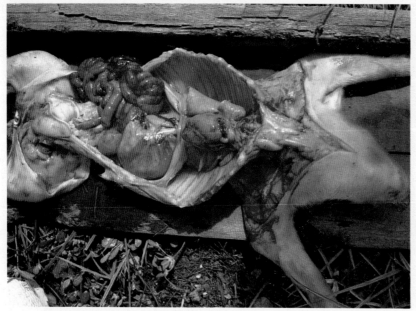

**Plates 283,284   Pig Enterotox-
emia**

There is severe reddening of the serosal
surfaces of the affected intestine. The
loops are filled with gas.   Clostridium
perfringens Type C is mostly isolated.

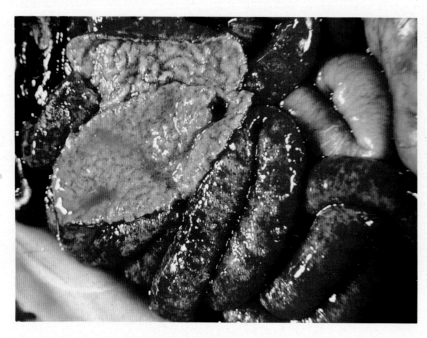

Plate 284   Pig Enterotoxemia

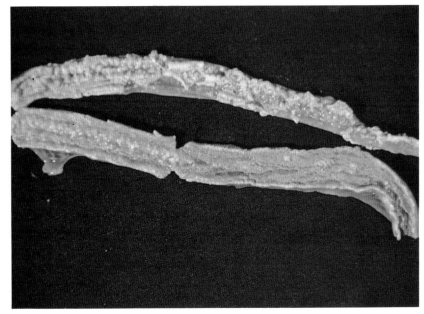

**Plates 285,286   Pig Enterotox-
emia**

In some instances a fibrinonecrotic enteritis develops.

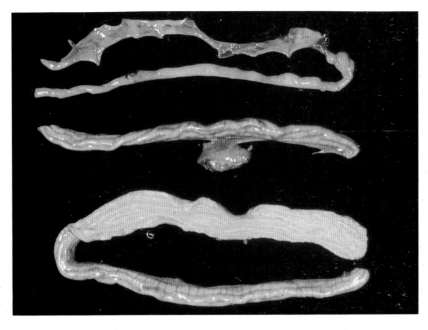

Plate 286   Pig Enterotoxemia

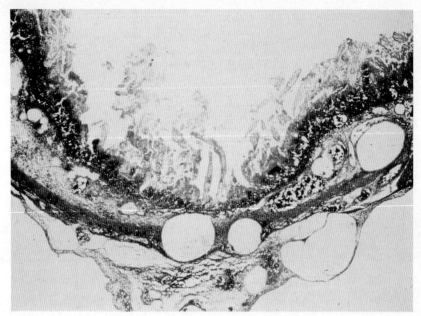

Plate 287　Pig Enterotoxemia
Histologically. severe necrosis and gas accumulation are present in the mucosa and submucosa. H&E stain.

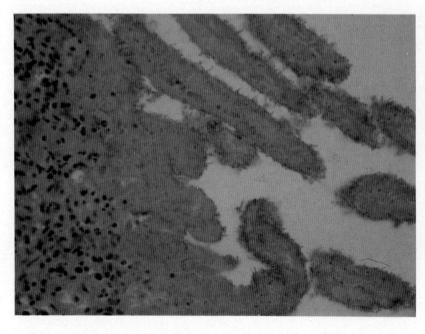

Plate 288　Pig Enterotoxemia
Numerous rod-shaped bacteria cover the mucosal surface. Gram stain.

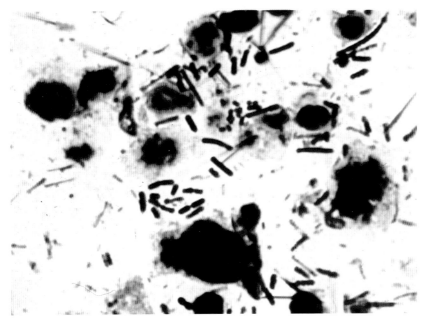

Plate 289   Pig Enterotoxemia

Scrapings from feces reveal a monotonous population of rods suggesting Clostridium perfringens.

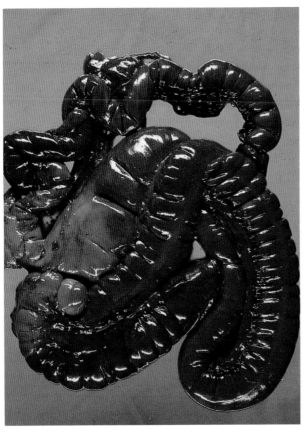

Plates 290,291   Equine Enterotoxemia

Clostridium perfringens type A is usually responsible for the severe edema and hemorrhagic suffusion of the intestinal wall of foals.

156

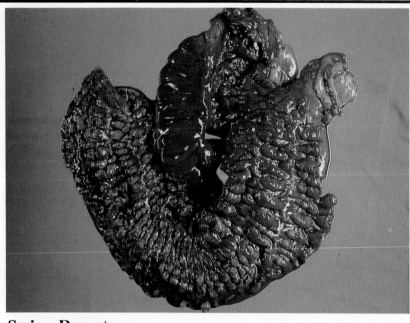

**Plate 291   Equine Enterotox-
emia**

Swine Dysentery

This disease is caused by a large spirochete known as Serpulina (Treponema) hyodysenteriae. Pigs 8-14 weeks are affected and develop "black scours". Anemia is a reliable clinical marker for swine dysentery. The inflammatory response is originally characterized by mucoid typhlocolitis. Later,superficial necrosis of the mucosa develops with erosions of blood vessels. The ileum becomes infected as well. Superimposed may be infections with Fusobacterium, Campylobacter and Salmonella spp.

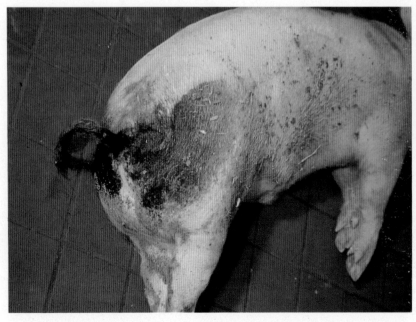

Plates 292,293   Swine Dysentery

Note generalized anemia and tarry, blood-stained feces around rump and tail. This is, however, not pathognomonic for swine dysentery. Feces are soft and blood-tinged.

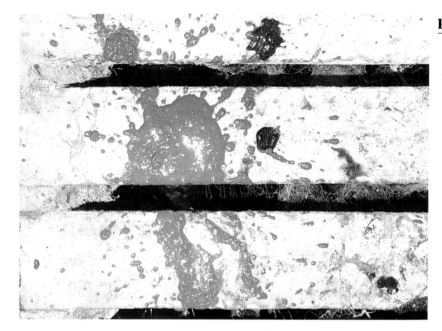

Plate 293   Swine Dysentery

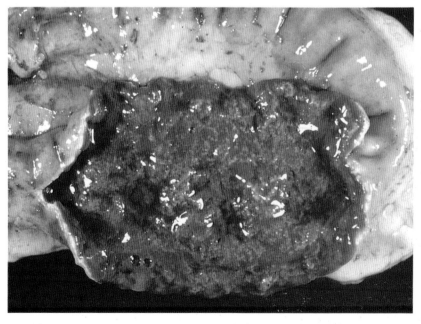

Plates 294-297   Swine Dysentery

Hemorrhagic and necrotic small and large intestine.   Pseudomembranes may develop in addition.

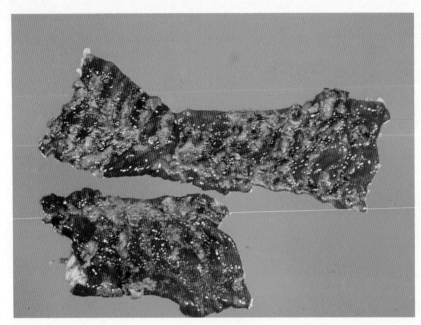

Plate 295   Swine Dysentery

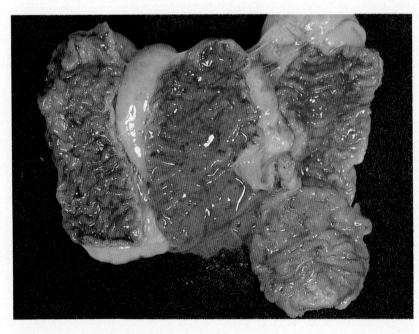

Plate 296   Swine Dysentery

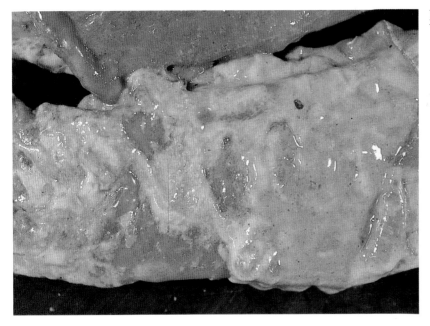

Plate 297　Swine Dysentery

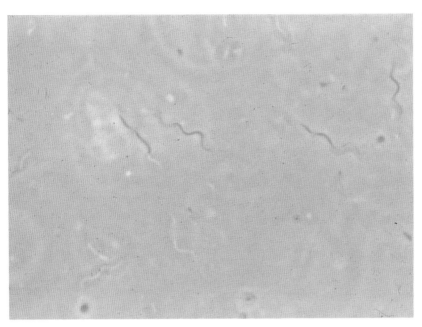

Plate 298　　Swine Dysentery
Dark-field microscopic examination of colonic epithelium scrapings demonstrates large coiled spirochetes.

Hemorrhagic Bowel Syndrome of Swine (Proliferative Enteritis) PHE

Pigs 1-10 months are affected. Depending on the morphologic presentation various names have been attached to the disease. The principal lesions are necrosis, hemorrhage, inflammation and hyperplasia of the ileum and sometimes cecum and colon. Brown, watery or hemorrhagic diarrhea are signs of the disease. The causative agent is thought to be Campylobacter hyointestinalis, a curved, rod-shaped intracellular organism. Recent antigenic and DNA analyses of the agent resulted in the recognition that the intracellular organism may be unrelated to Campylobacter sp.

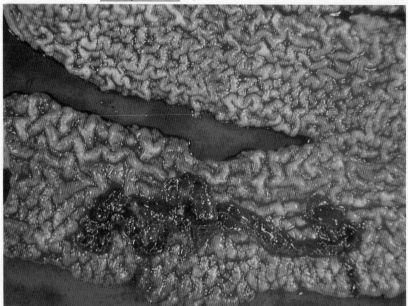

Plate 299   PHE

A large blood clot is present in the opened lumen of a very thickened ileum.

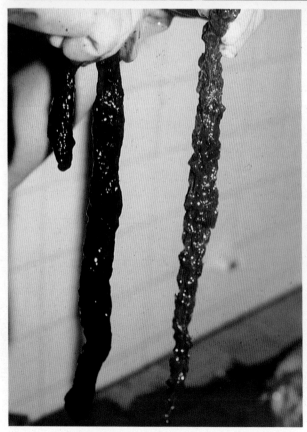

Plate 300   PHE

Blood clots are passed with feces.

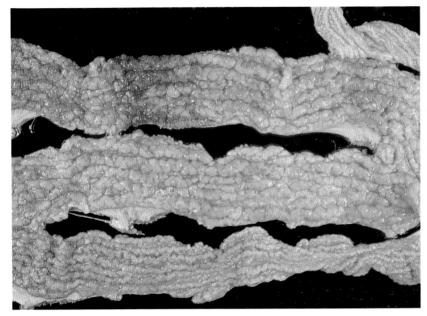

Plate 301 PHE

Marked diffuse mucosal corrugation characterizes the chronic form of PHE.

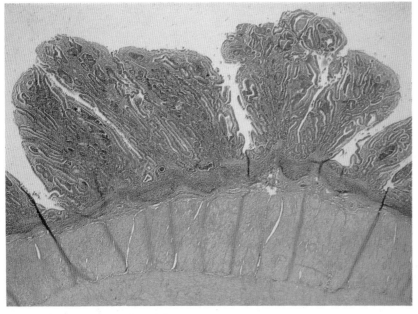

Plates 302,303 PHE

Microscopically, there is marked proliferation of mucosal epithelium with a nodular, adenomatous pattern. The epithelial cells vary from cuboidal to columnar. The lamina propria is mildly infiltrated with lymphocytes.

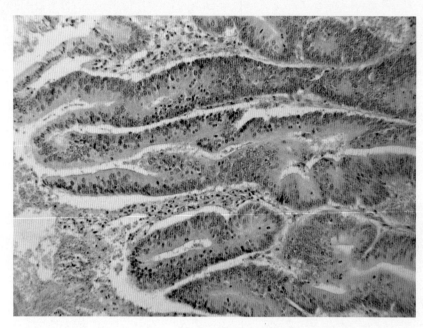

Plate 303   PHE

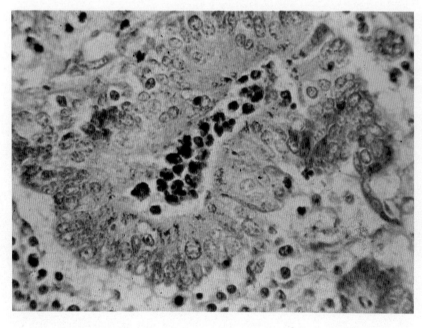

Plate 304   PHE

Campylobacter sp. are microaerophilic and can be demonstrated with silver stains as small intracellular organisms. GMS stain.

Colitis X of Horses

This highly fatal peracute disease of horses is characterized by explosive, copious, watery diarrhea. The cause remains unclear, but is attributed to endotoxic shock, salmonellosis or clostridial disease. The fatal outcome is the result of cardiovascular collapse.

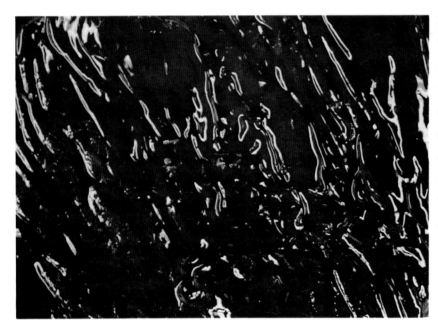

Plates 305,306   Colitis X

The colon appears markedly edematous, and the deep blue color is the result of venous congestion and blockage. Most cases of acute colitis are preceded by stress such as performance, exhibition, shipping, surgery. Horses of all ages may be affected. The large bowel has been proposed as being the shock organ of the horse.

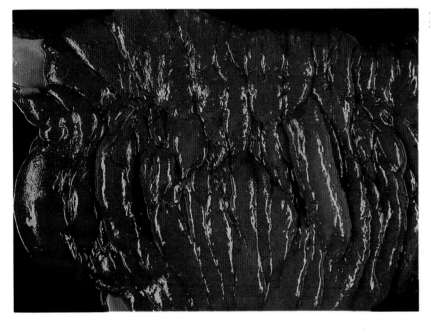

Plate 306   Colitis X

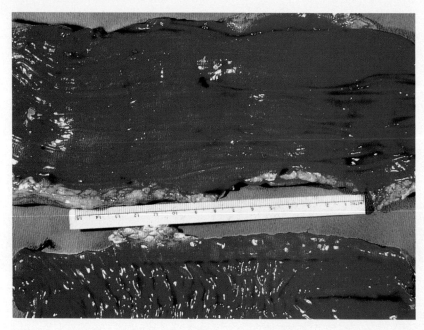

Plate 307　Intestinal Toxins

Ingestion of toxins has to be considered in the differential diagnosis of hemorrhagic enteritis. This is arsenic toxicosis in a bovine. Oleander can cause a similar enteric condition.

(d)　Fibrinous Enteritis
　　Feline Panleukopenia

This highly fatal parvovirus mainly affects the small intestine of cats. The virus attacks the cryptal cells.

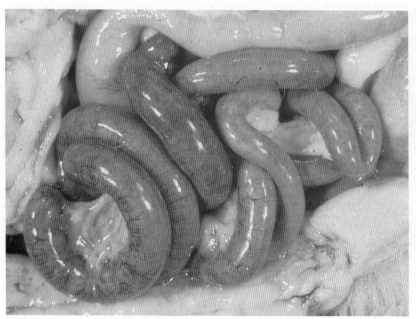

Plate 308　Feline Panleukopenia

Hyperemic. dilated. flaccid segments of jejunum and ileum in feline panleukopenia. Other portions of the serosa have a ground-glass appearance. The lesion can be segmental at the gross level.

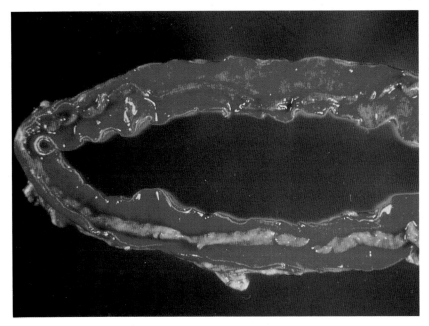

Plate 309 Feline Panleukopenia

Formation of fibrin casts in jejunum. Note hemorrhagic appearance of mucosa.

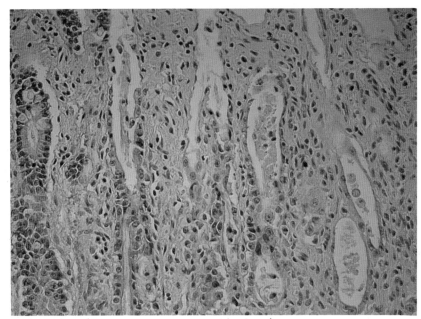

Plates 310,311 Feline Panleukopenia

Microscopically, the villus stroma is collapsed and condensed. In the basal portion of the mucosa, the crypts are dilated by seromucinous fluid. Degenerated epithelial cells are desquamated into the dilated crypts. Regeneration of damaged cryptal epithelium or proliferation of unaffected epithelial cells may occur. Intranuclear inclusion bodies may be demonstrated in specially fixed, fresh intestinal tissues in the very early phases of the disease.

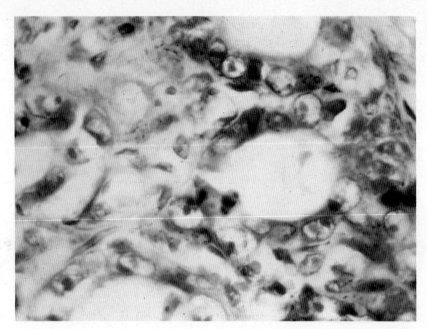

Plate 311　Feline　Panleukopenia

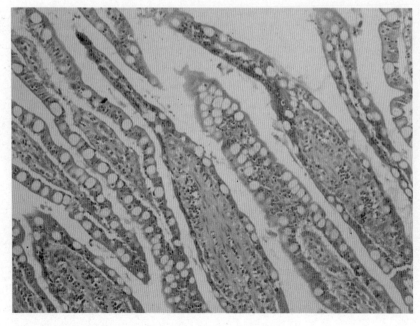

Plate 312 Feline Colostrum Globules

Colostrum absorbing enterocytes should not be confused with degenerative changes associated with feline panleukopenia.

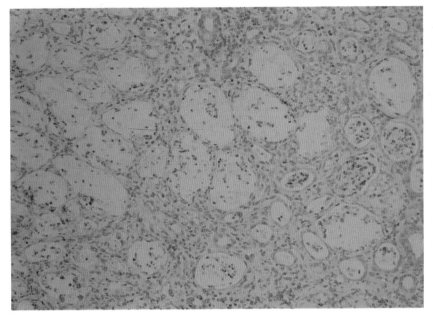

Plate 313   Feline Colitis

Cases of desquamative cryptitis in the colon may be the result of infection with FeLV virus.

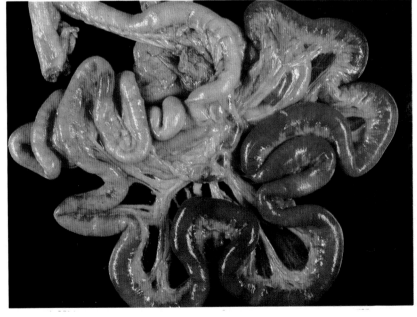

Plates 314-317   Canine Parvovirus

In the 1970's, outbreaks of severe diarrheal diseases in young purebred dogs were the result of infection with the canine parvovirus. Major clinical signs included vomiting and hemorrhagic diarrhea. The gross changes are characterized by dark, red to purple discoloration of the serosal and mucosal surfaces of the small intestinal tract. Luminal contents are liquid and red. The mesenteric lymph nodes are reddened and enlarged. Intussusception may occur from dysperistalsis.

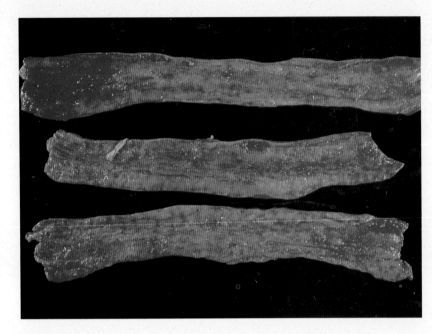

Plate 315   Canine Parvovirus

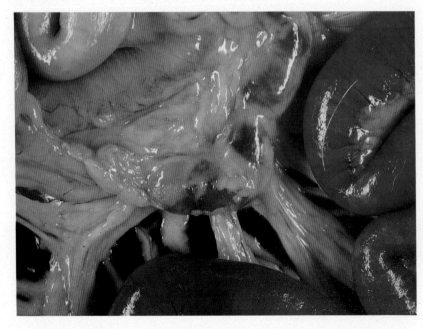

Plate 316   Canine Parvovirus

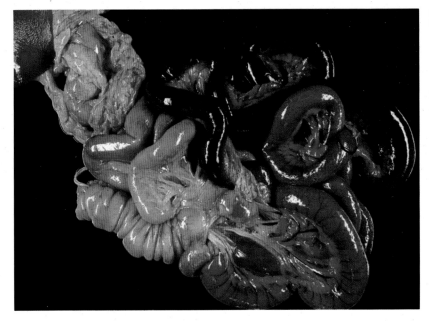

Plate 317   Canine Parvovirus

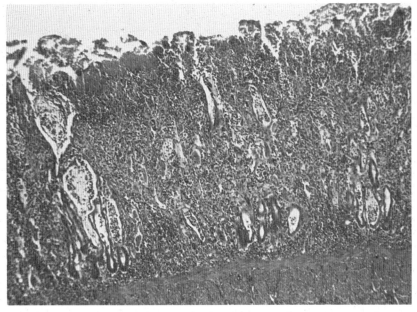

Plates 318-319   Canine Parvovirus

Necrosis of the cryptal epithelium is the characteristic morphologic feature of this canine viral infection.   There is loss of epithelial cells with dilatation of remaining crypts. In more advanced cases, there is regeneration of cryptal epithelium as demonstrated here. The lesions are remarkably similar to those of feline panleukopenia.

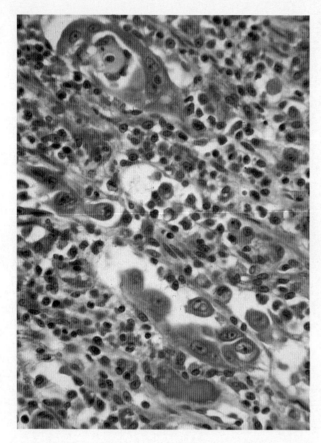

Plate 319   Canine Parvovirus

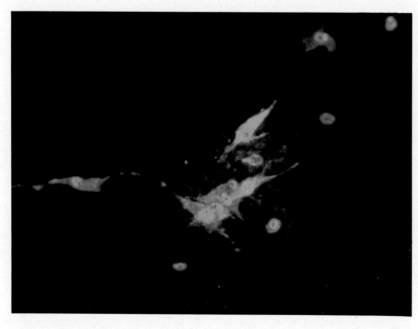

Plates 320,321 Canine Parvovirus

Virus can be demonstrated with fluorescence technique in tissue or from feces under the electron microscope.

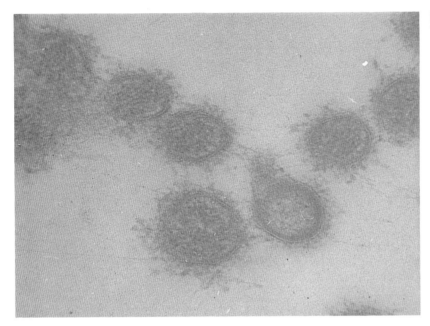

Plate 321   Canine Parvovirus

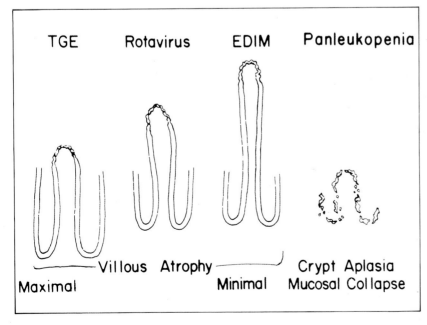

Plate 322   Enteric Viruses

The diagram outlines the development of intestinal lesions caused by some enteric viruses. (Reproduced by permission of the Journal of the American Veterinary Medical Association.)

Salmonellosis

Young animals have a greater susceptibility to infection with Salmonella sp. than adult animals. Adults may be carriers. The bacilli produce endotoxins. There are acute or chronic forms of salmonellosis. Salmonella sp. in the acute disease phase cause catarrhal or hemorrhagic enteritis. Later on, the mucosa becomes necrotic and sloughs forming casts in the lumen. Crusty, scabby mucosal changes characterize the chronic forms.

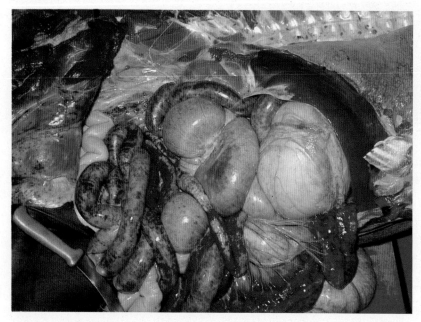

Plates 323-325   Equine Salmonellosis

This is septicemic salmonellosis in a foal. The intestinal serosa is deeply red; the mucosa shows early pseudomembrane formation.

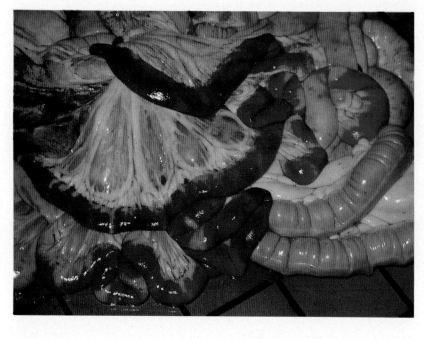

Plate 324   Equine Salmonellosis

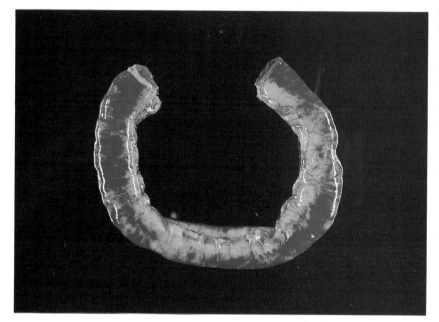

Plate 325   Equine Salmonellosis

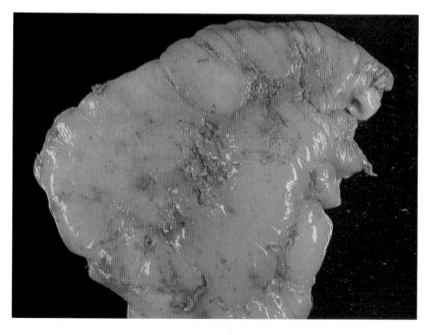

**Plates 326–328   Equine Salmo-
nellosis**

Acute salmonellosis in the large colon of
an adult horse. Note edema and congestion of the mucosa and submucosa suggesting severe vascular compromise.

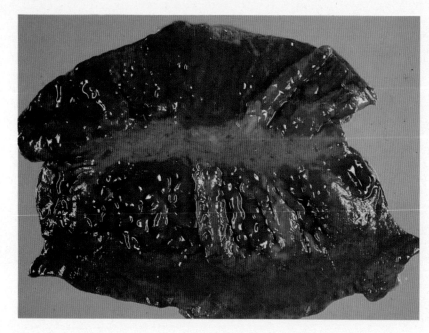

Plate 327   Equine Salmonellosis

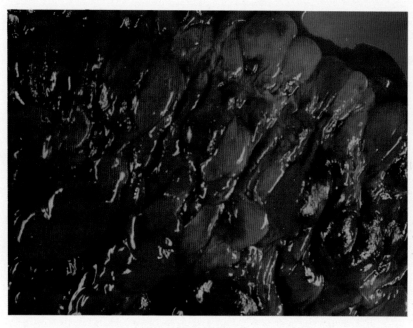

Plate 328   Equine Salmonellosis

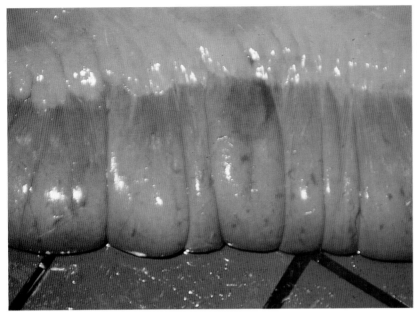

Plate 329   Equine Salmonellosis

In some cases the vascular thrombosis involves all intramural blood vessels.

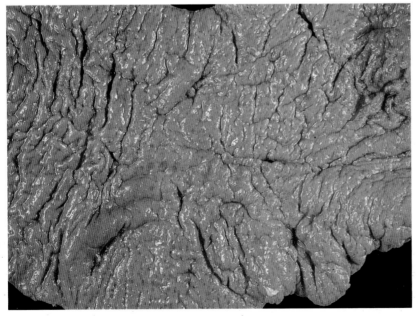

Plates 330-332   Equine Salmonellosis

Chronic salmonellosis is characterized by leathery thickening of the mucosa and lymphadenopathy of draining lymph nodes.

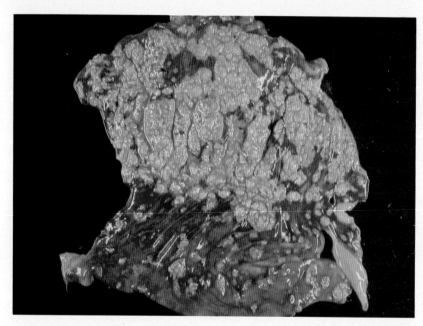

Plate 331   Equine Salmonellosis

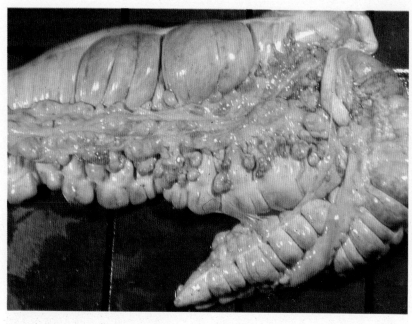

Plate 332   Equine Salmonellosis

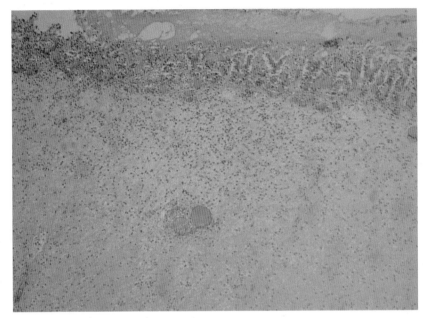

**Plates 333-335 Equine Salmo-
nellosis**

Microscopic findings of edema, hemorrhage, congestion and thrombosis are indicators of endotoxic shock. H&E stain.

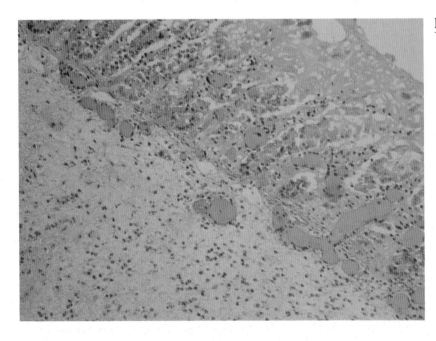

Plate 334 Equine Salmonellosis

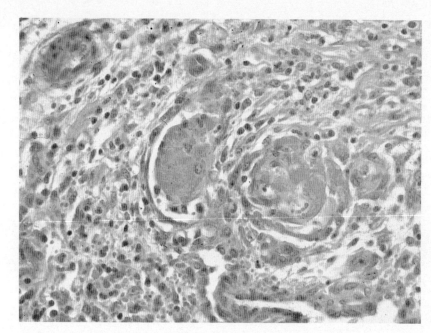

Plate 335   Equine Salmonellosis

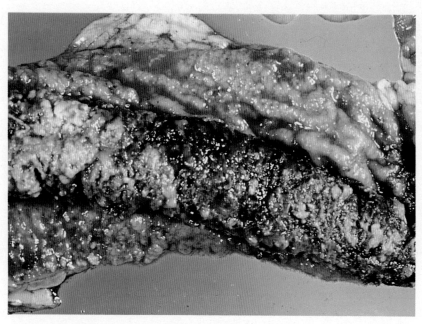

Plate 336   Bovine Salmonellosis
Ileum of a cow with chronic salmonellosis.
S. typhimurium was isolated. Note fibrinonecrotic casts and the formation of pseudomembranes on the mucosa.

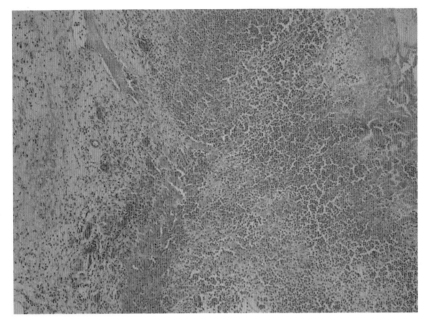

Plates 337,338   Bovine Salmonellosis

Fibrin and degenerating neutrophils. H&E stain.

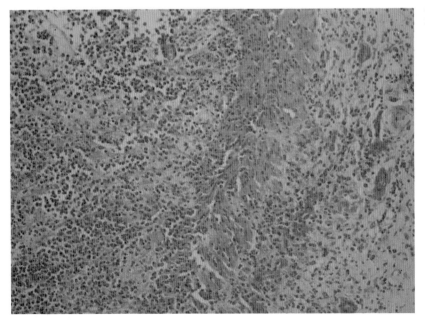

Plate 338   Bovine Salmonellosis

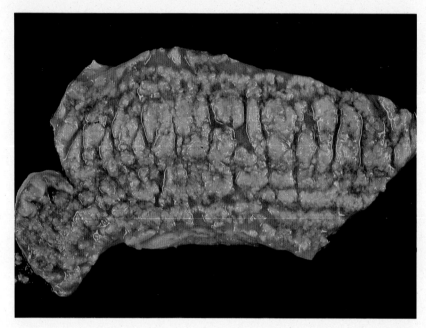

Plate 339 Bovine Salmonellosis
Chronic salmonellosis is characterized by thick mucosal crusts.

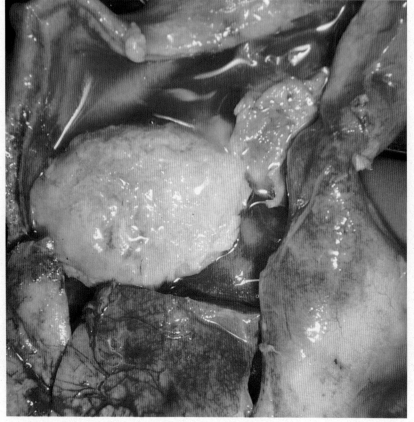

Plate 340 Bovine Salmonellosis
In calves, circumstantial evidence for the diagnosis of Salmonella infection is the finding of fibrin casts in the gallbladder. (arrow)

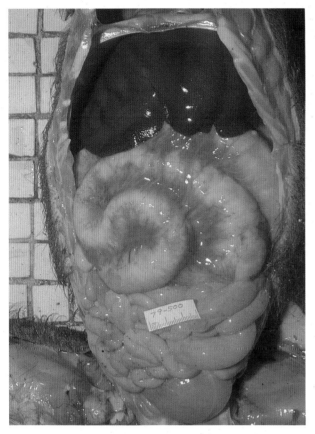

Plate 341   Porcine Salmonellosis

Markedly distended intestinal tract in a sow with early peritonitis.

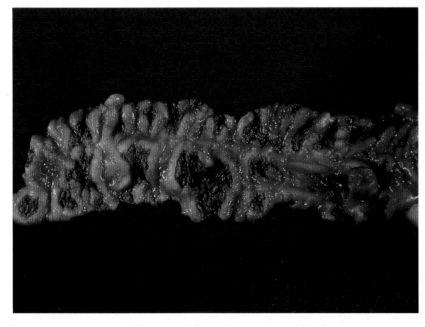

Plates 342-347   Porcine Salmonellosis

Intestine with fibrinonecrotic and ulcerative colitis. In the pig, Salmonella typhimurium and Salmonella cholerae-suis are the most frequent isolates. Enteritis, septicemia and bacteremia are common features. Liver and lung frequently are involved in showing evidence of septicemia.

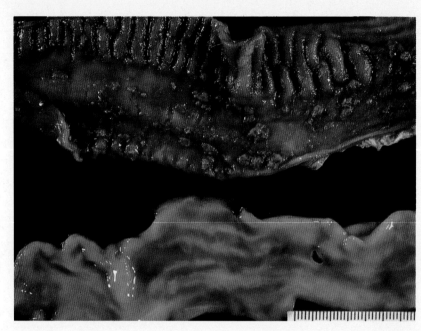

Plate 343   **Porcine Salmonellosis**

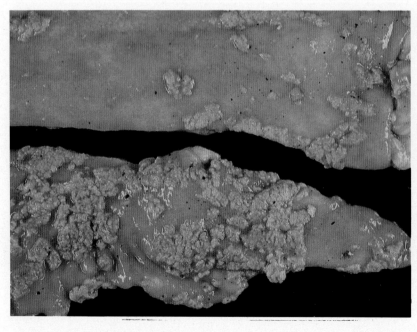

Plate 344   **Porcine Salmonellosis**

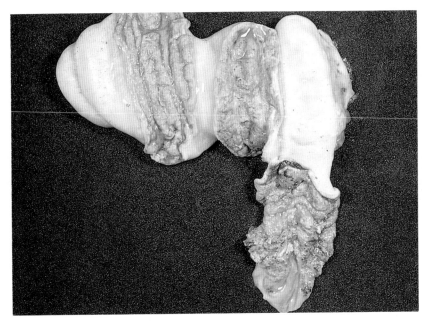

Plate 345   Porcine Salmonel-
losis

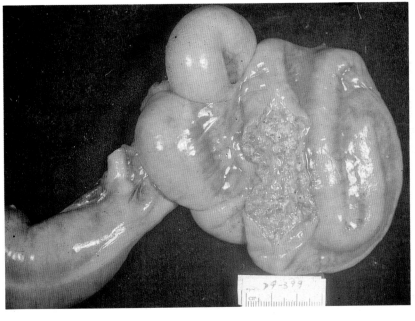

Plate 346   Porcine Salmonel-
losis

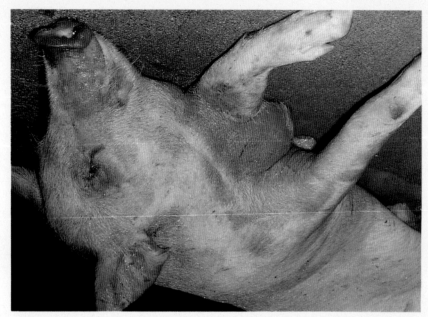

Plate 347   Porcine Salmonellosis

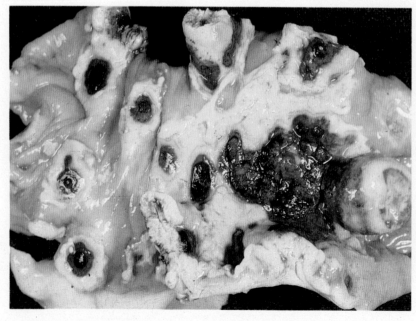

Plate 348   Porcine Salmonellosis

The "button ulcers" in the colon of a pig are caused by S. cholerae-suis, but also may be seen in pigs with hog cholera.

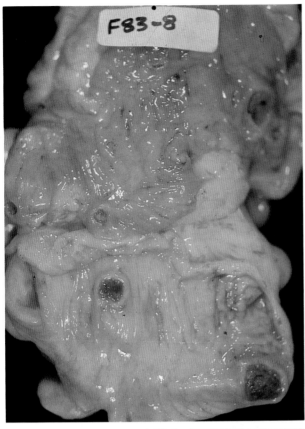

Plates 349,350   Intestinal Hog Cholera

"Button ulcer" formation in this viral disease should be differentiated from salmonellosis.   There also is evidence of transmural hemorrhage.

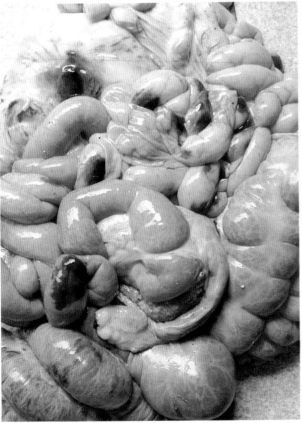

Plate 350   Intestinal Hog Cholera

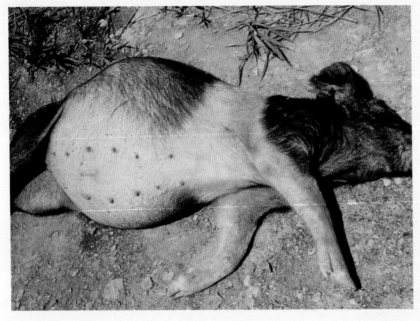

Plates 351–354 Rectal Stricture

It has been suggested that S. typhimurium is involved in the pathogenesis of this syndrome in younger pigs. The evidence may be circumstantial and the isolation may be secondary to the severe impaction and stasis of feces in the terminal colon of pigs. Others have suggested that genetic factors are associated with the development of rectal strictures. The stricture site typically is very close to the anus, severely distends the spiral colon of affected pigs and can cause peritonitis in advanced cases.

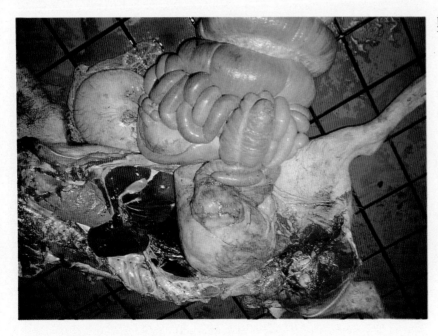

Plate 352 Rectal Stricture

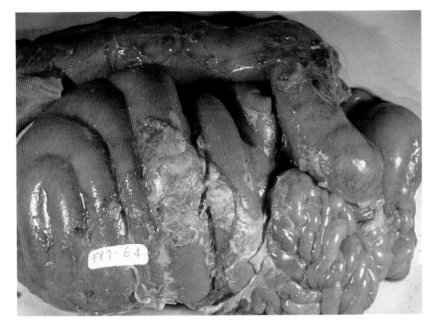

Plate 353   Rectal Stricture

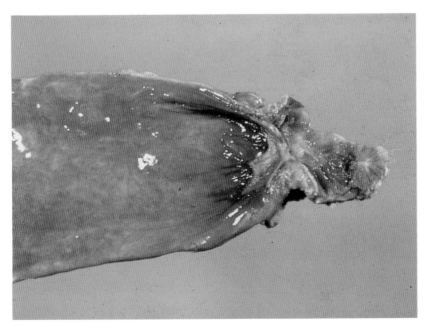

Plate 354   Rectal Stricture

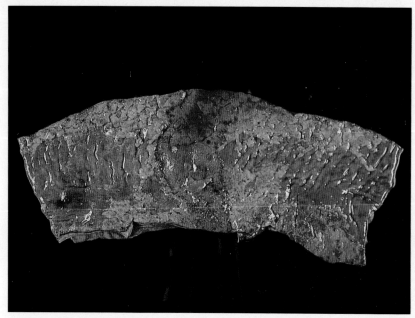

Plate 355 Intestinal Toxicosis

Toxins with caustic effects should be considered as differential diagnosis for fibrinous enteritis. This is Quercus (oak) toxicosis of the jejunum in a cow.

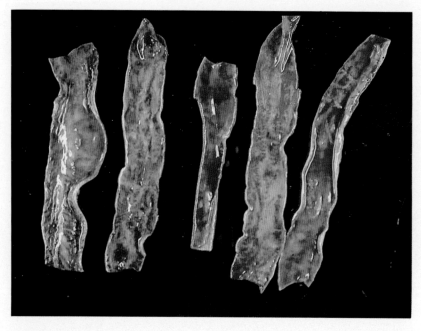

Plate 356 Radiation

Radiation may cause fibrinous enteritis as illustrated in a dog.

(e) Ulcerative - Necrotizing Enteritis

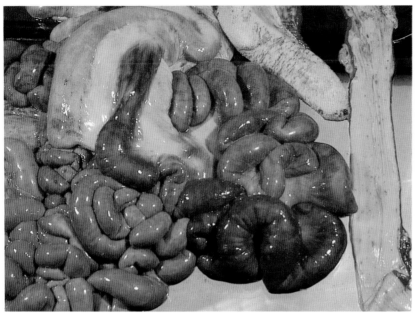

Plate 357　BVD

Cattle infected with the BVD virus develop hemorrhagic, necrotizing enteritis in the small intestine.

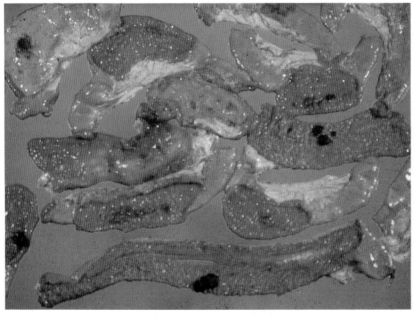

Plates 358,359　BVD

Necrosis of Peyer's patches is a typical finding in cattle infected with the bovine virus diarrhea virus.

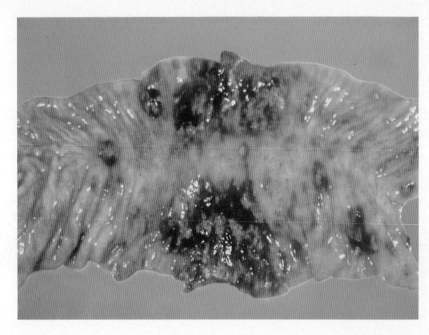

Plate 359   BVD

Plate 360 Salmonellosis

In bovine Salmonella infection similar changes can occur in the Peyer's patches.

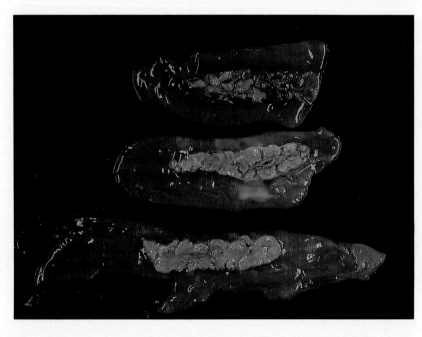

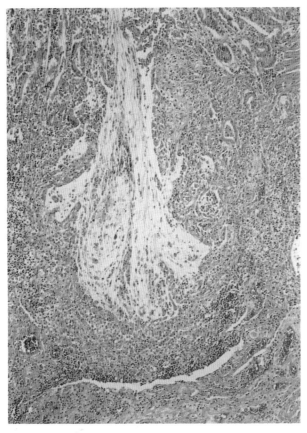

Plate 361　BVD

Microscopically, lymphoid follicles show necrosis of lymphocytes in BVD.　H&E stain.

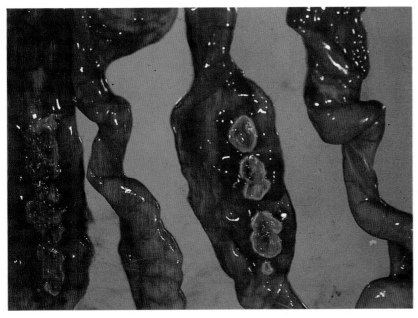

Plates 362,363　　Mycotic Enteritis

The intestinal tract is rather resistent to infection with fungi. These are sporadic examples of mycotic ulcers in the ileum of a calf and colon of a cat.

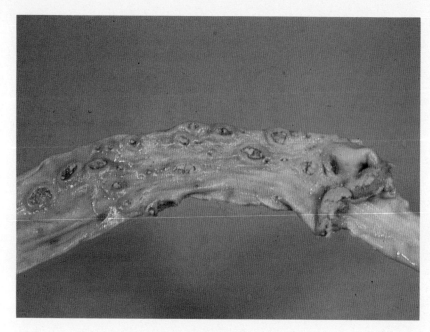

Plate 363   Mycotic Enteritis

Potomac Horse Fever (PHF)

Potomac horse fever (equine ehrlichial colitis) is a disease of horses that originally was identified in regions adjacent to the Potomac River in Virginia and Maryland.   It now has spread throughout the eastern coast of the US.PHF is characterized by fever, anorexia, leukopenia, diarrhea and dehydration.   Case fatality rate may be as high as 30%.   The disease affects the large colon of horses. The causative agent is Ehrlichia risticii.   The organism can be demonstrated by silver stains or electronmicroscopy.

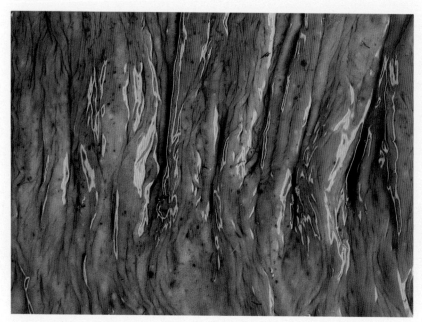

Plate 364   PHF

Grossly, shallow red erosions are visible in the large colon of an affected horse.

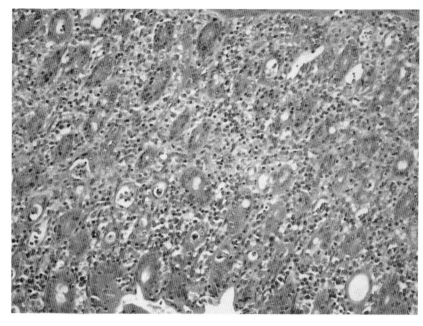

Plate 365 PHF

Histologically, a mixed inflammation is visible in the mucosa. Intracytoplasmic organisms can be present within both glandular epithelial cells and macrophages. Organisms also can be detected in blood leukocytes. H&E stain.

(f) Purulent Enteritis

Neutrophils are the predominant inflammatory cells in this type of enteritis. Abscesses form within crypts. Primate shigellosis is a good disease example.

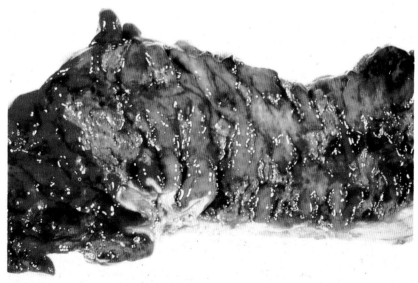

Plates 366,367   Shigellosis

The disease is caused by Shigella flexneri and occurs in monkeys that have been stressed. The disease is clinically characterized by watery, mucinous diarrhea mixed with blood. Gross findings include diffuse or patchy areas of hemorrhage. Ulcers may or may not be present. The pathologic changes usually are confined to the colon. Infection with Pseudomonas aeruginosa may create similar gross findings in monkeys.

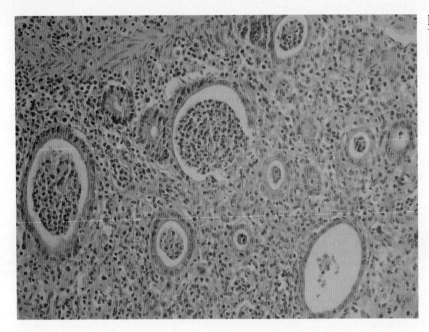

Plate 367   Shigellosis

(g) Chronic Granulomatous Proliferative Diseases

Chronic inflammatory processes affecting the intestinal tract are associated with malassimilation and chronic diarrhea.   Maldigestion, malabsorption through inadequate absorptive surfaces, biochemical defects in transport, chronic inflammatory infiltrates within the intestinal wall and defects in the flow of intestinal lymph are causes of the malassimilation syndrome.

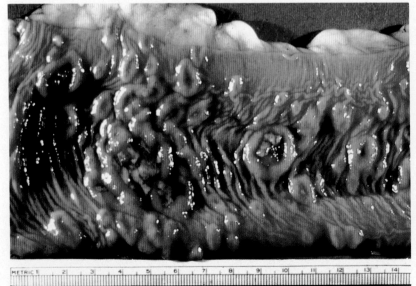

Plate 368   Intestinal Tuberculosis

Pathogenic mycobacteria are the cause of mammalian tuberculosis. The jejunum of a cow is affected by the mammalian type of mycobacteriosis. Notice the focal mucosal elevations with central ulcers.

Paratuberculosis (Johne's Disease)

Mycobacterium paratuberculosis is the causative agent. All ruminants are naturally susceptible to the bacillus. Clinical signs include persistent diarrhea and weight loss despite a good appetite. The small intestinal tract is the usual target organ for the bacilli and for pathological changes to occur. These are featured by mucosal thickening, lymphangiectasia and lymphadenopathy of draining mesenteric lymph nodes. Histologically, the intestinal wall and mesenteric lymph nodes are infiltrated with macrophages (epithelioid cells) and giant cells of Langhans' type.

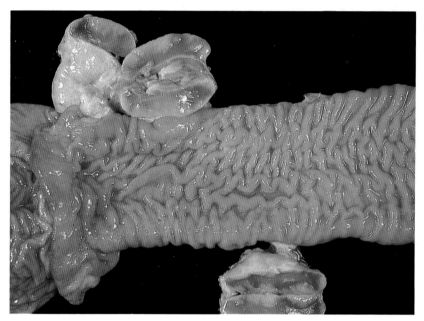

Plate 369   Bovine Paratuberculosis

The lesions of paratuberculosis develop most consistently in the terminal ileum. The intestinal mucosa is uniformly thickened and thrown into transverse rugae which will not disappear when the intestinal tract is stretched. Ulceration is not a feature in cattle with paratuberculosis. Adjacent lymph nodes are enlarged.

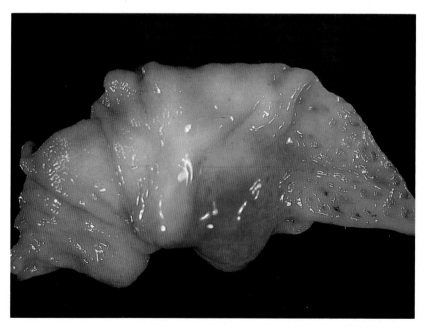

Plate 370   Bovine Paratuberculosis

Thickening and reddening of the ileo-cecal valve can occur.

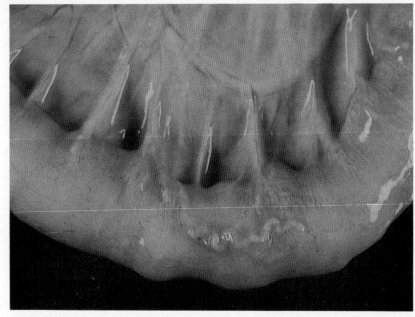

Plate 371 Bovine Paratuberculosis

Subserosal lymphatics are distended and beaded.

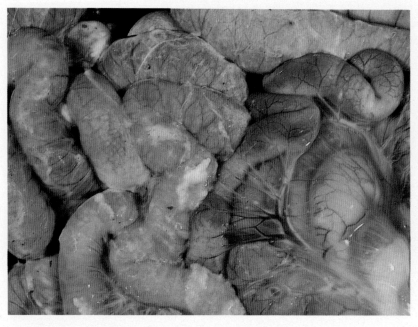

Plates 372,373 Ovine Paratuberculosis

In small ruminants. the mucosal corrugation frequently is not obvious. Transmural inflammation is characterized by white nodules. and mesenteric lymphatics are distended.

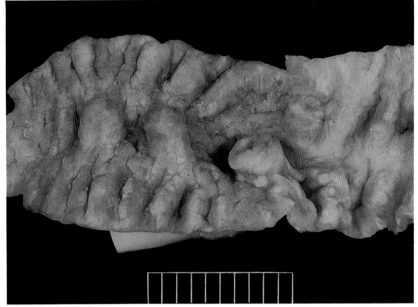

**Plate 373   Ovine Paratuberculo-
sis**

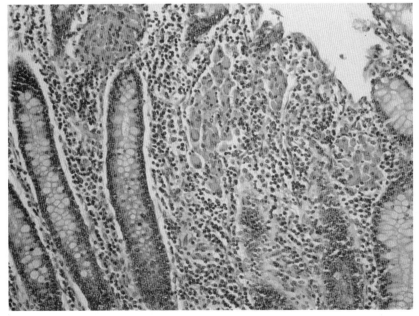

**Plates 374,375   Paratubercu-
losis**
Microscopically, the mucosa and submucosa are markedly infiltrated by epithelioid cells and occasional Langhans' type
giant cells. H&E stain.

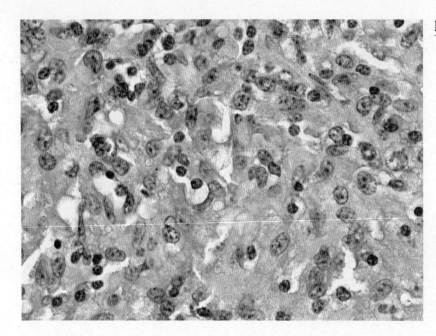

Plate 375   Paratuberculosis

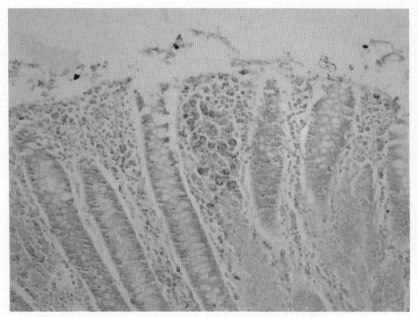

Plates 376,377   Paratuberculosis

Special stains readily demonstrate numerous, clustered, intracellular acid-fast mycobacteria in paratuberculosis. Ziehl-Neelsen stain.

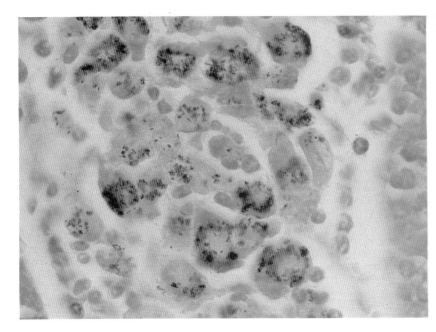

Plate 377   **Paratuberculosis**

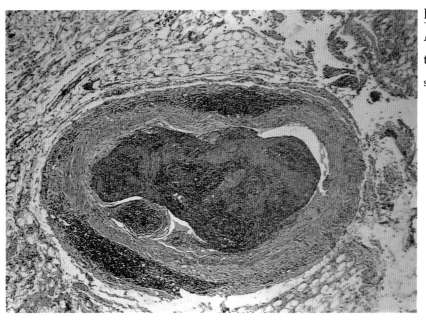

Plate 378   **Paratuberculosis**

A granulomatous endo- and perilymphangitis are responsible for the grossly observed lymphatic distention.   H&E stain.

Equine Granulomatous Enteritis of Known Etiology

Recently reported cases of chronic granulomatous enteritis in the horse were associated with malabsorption and hypoproteinemia. The thickening and granular appearance of the ileal mucosa resembled bovine paratuberculosis. In addition, ulcers developed in the large colon, a feature which is not typical of Johne's disease. Histologically, the intestinal wall was diffusely infiltrated by macrophages, eosinophils and inflammatory giant cells. Etiologic agents were identified in a few of the cases. These were Mycobacterium avium-intracellulare, Rhodococcus equi and Histoplasma capsulatum.

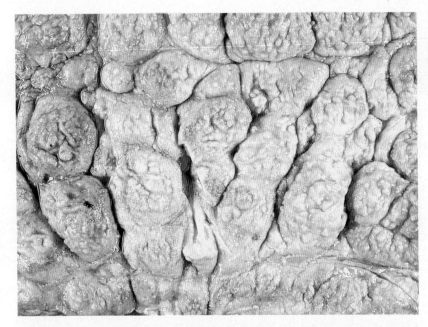

Plate 379 Intestinal Equine Mycobacteriosis

Thickening and ulceration of large colon mucosa in horse with M. avium infection.

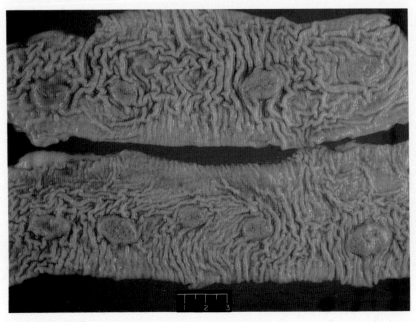

Plate 380 Intestinal Equine Mycobacteriosis

Ileum with prominent lymphoid nodules (Peyer's patches)

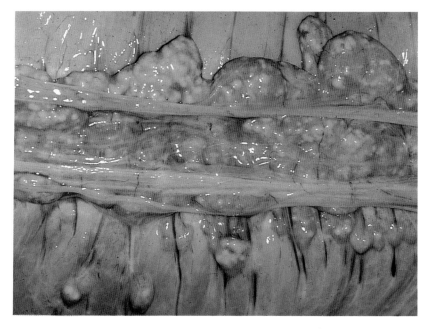

Plates 381,382 Intestinal Equine Mycobacteriosis

Colonic and mesenteric lymph nodes are markedly enlarged.

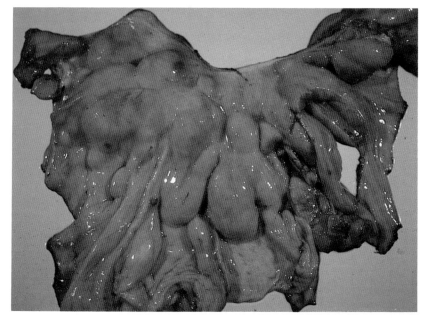

Plate 382 Intestinal Equine Mycobacteriosis

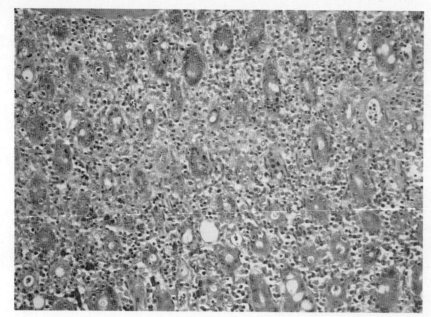

Plates 383,384 Intestinal Equine Mycobacteriosis

Microscopically, the lamina propria of the colon is diffusely and markedly infiltrated by epithelioid macrophages and some lymphocytes. H&E stain.

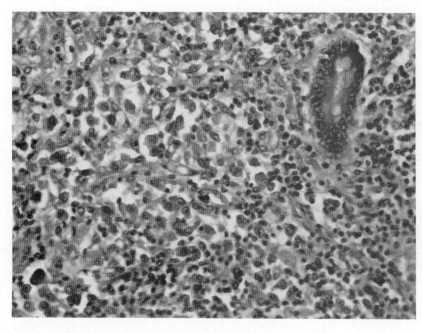

Plate 384 Intestinal Equine Mycobacteriosis

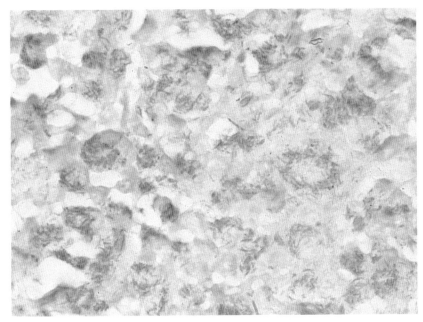

Plate 385　Intestinal Equine My-cobacteriosis

Epithelioid macrophages are filled with myriads of intracellular, acid-fast bacilli. Ziehl-Neelsen stain.

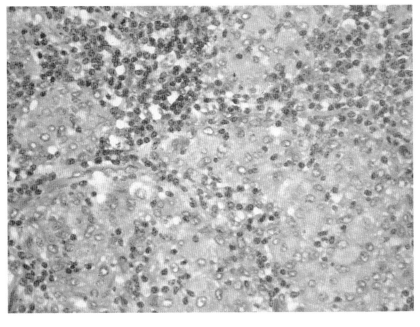

Plate 386　Intestinal Equine My-cobacteriosis

Epithelioid macrophages have drained into regional lymph nodes. H&E stain.

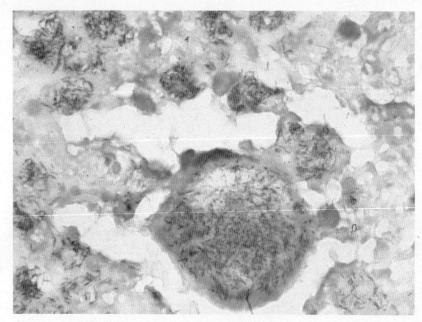

Plate 387 Intestinal Equine My-cobacteriosis

Nodal epithelioid macrophages are packed with acid-fast bacilli. Ziehl-Neelsen stain.

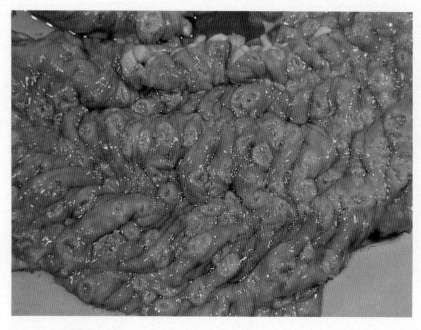

Plate 388   Intestinal Histoplasmosis

This corrugated, thickened mucosa of equine large colon is infected with Histoplasma capsulatum. Many small ulcers with irregular edges are visible.

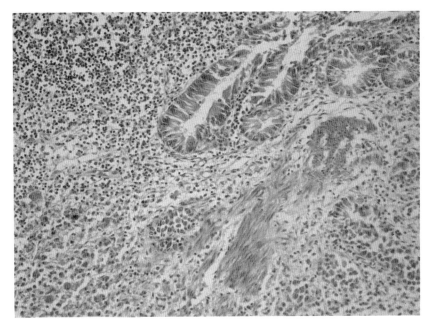

Plate 389   Intestinal Histoplas-mosis

Microscopically, portions of the mucosa are infiltrated with macrophages, lympho-cytes and plasma cells.   H&E stain.

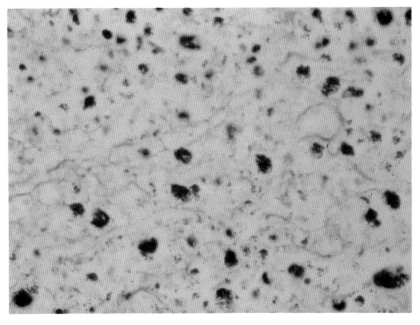

Plate 390   Intestinal Histoplas-mosis

The macrophages contain numerous yeast-like bodies in the cytoplasm as demon-strated with this silver stain.   Warthy-Starry stain.

Intestinal Rhodococcus Equi Infection

Young horses, especially those that are immunologically compromised may develop the intestinal form of Rhodococcus equi infection. The infection may be ulcerative or proliferative.

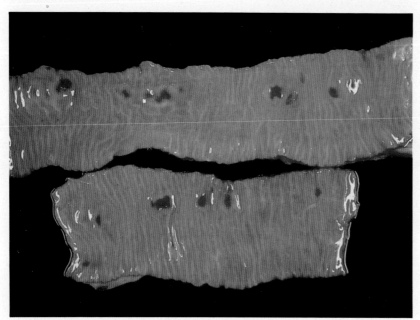

Plate 391   R. equi

Ulcerative changes are present in the ileum of a young horse infected with R. equi.

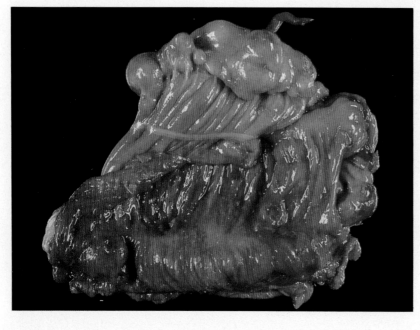

Plate 392   R. equi

The colon shows a more diffuse, erosive, necrotizing form of inflammation.

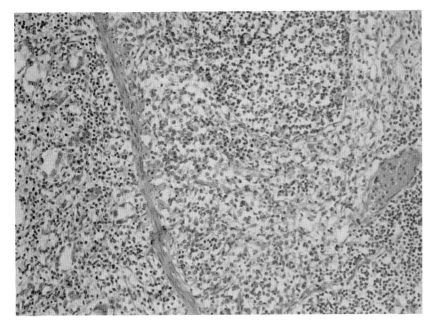

Plates 393,394 R. equi

Microscopically, the lamina propria diffusely is infiltrated by macrophages. Necrosis of lymphoid follicles and mucosal epithelial cells is an additional finding. H&E stain.

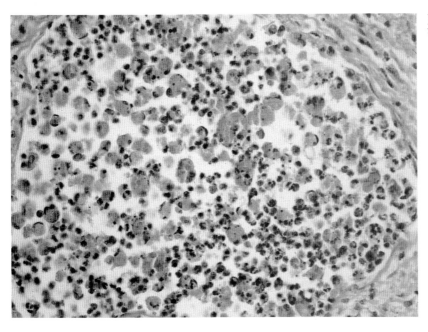

Plate 394 R. equi

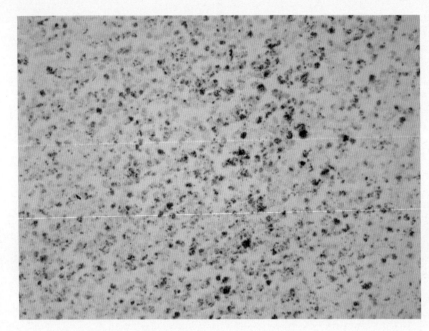

Plates 395,396   R. equi

A gram stain demonstrates numerous small intracellular gram-positive rods. Brown & Brenn stain.

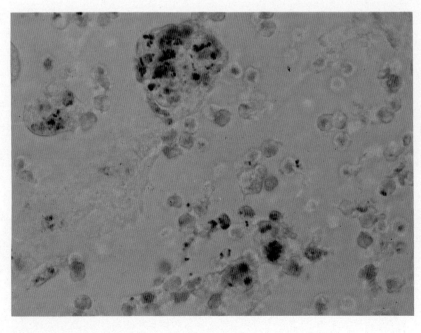

Plate 396   R. equi

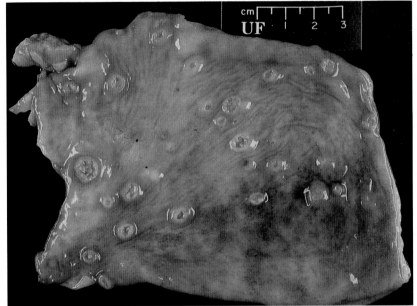

Plates 397 – 399   R. equi

More chronic cases of R. equi infection are featured by proliferative and ulcerative changes in the mucosa and submucosa as well as by enlarged draining lymph nodes.

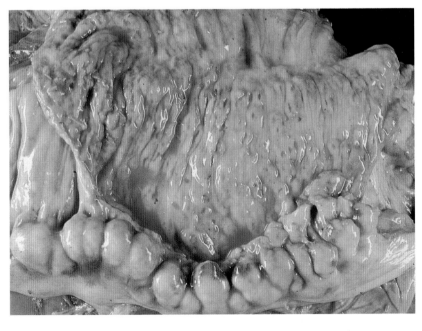

Plate 398   R. equi

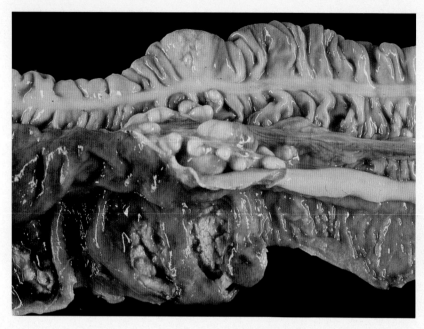

Plate 399   R. equi

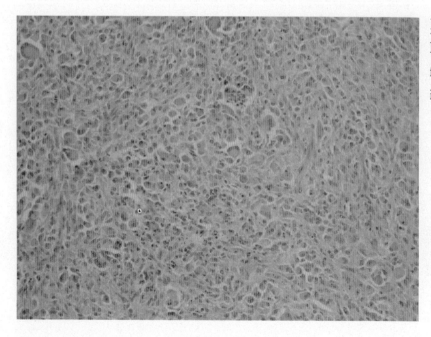

Plates 400   R. equi
Bizarre macrophages have infiltrated and filled the submucosa of a young horse infected with Rhodococcus equi.

Canine Histiocytic Ulcerative Colitis (CHUC)

This familial disease of young Boxer dogs is clinically associated with weight loss and diarrhea. The precise nature of its cause is undetermined.

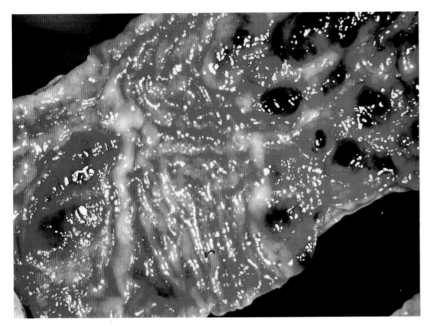

Plate 401   CHUC

Colon of Boxer dog is thickened, and the mucosa is ulcerated with clotted blood covering the denuded surface.

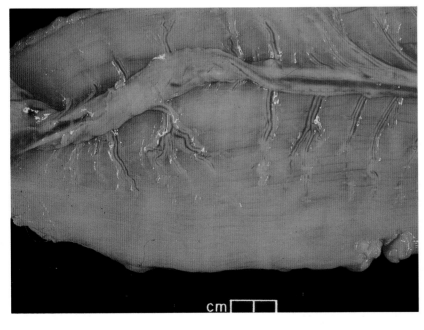

Plate 402   CHUC

In some cases inflammatory plaques occur on the serosal surface of the affected colon. These segments are indicative of transmural inflammation leading to deep sclerosis and adhesions.

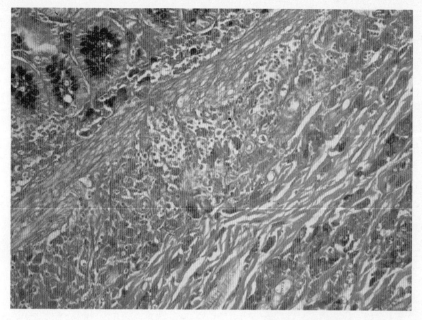

Plates 403,404   CHUC

Histologically, the mucosa and portions of the lamina propria are infiltrated by macrophages which have a pink. foamy cytoplasm. The cytoplasm stains positive for mucopolysaccharides. Notice the intensity of the stain when compared with the goblet cells in the mucosa. PAS stain.

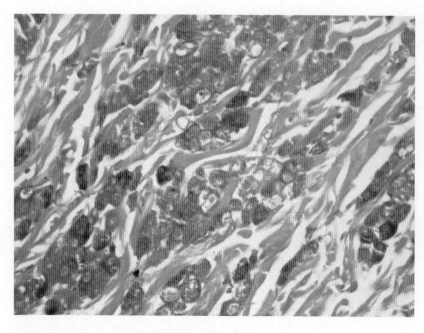

Plate 404   CHUC

Transmissible Ileal Hyperplasia of Hamsters (TIHH)

This disease also is known as "wet tail" or proliferative ileitis of hamsters. It is associated with scours. The ileum and occasionally the colon are affected. There is evidence of necrosis with regenerative hyperplasia of the mucosa. The disease originally thought to be caused by Campylobacter sp. is now believed to be associated with a slightly curved, gram-negative bacillus which may not be a member of the genus Campylobacter.

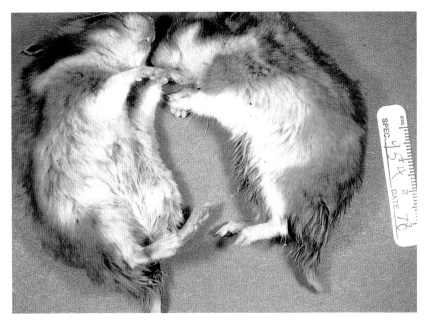

Plate 405   TIHH
Diarrhea staining the anus, tail and ventral abdomen of a hamster with TIHH.

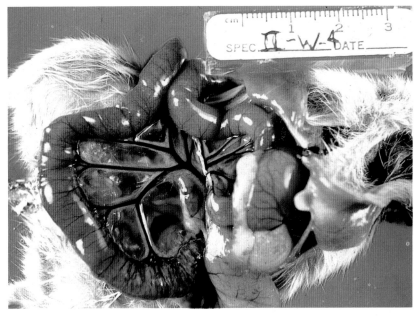

Plates 406   TIHH
The entire intestinal tract is distended due most likely to ileus.

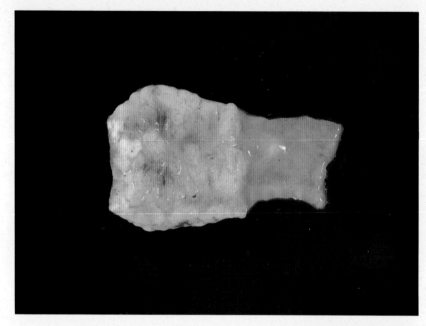

Plates 407,408   TIHH

The ileum is thickened and enlarged as
the result of pyogranulomatous inflammation and mucosal hyperplasia. The serosal
surface has a red hue and contains gray,
white nodules. Normal hamster ileum is
included. (From Jacoby R.O. Transmissible Ileal Hyperplasia of Hamsters.   I.
Histogenesis and Immunocytochemistry.
Am. J. Pathol. 91:445, 1978.)

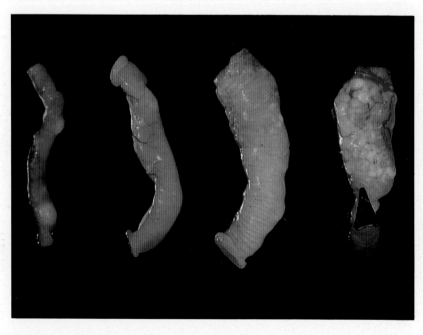

Plate 408   TIHH

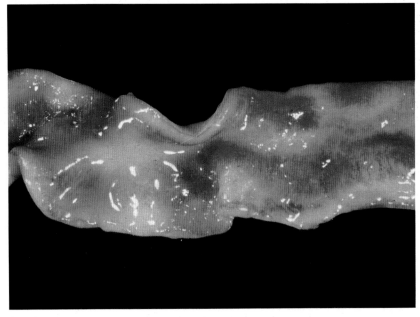

Plate 409   Ferret Campylobac-teriosis

Ileal lesion viewed from the luminal sur-face. Mucosal thickening is rather promi-nent and diffuse.

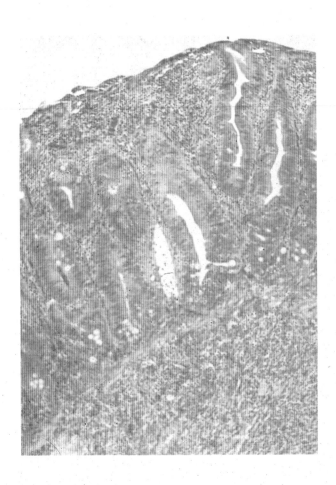

Plate 410   Ferret Campylobacte-riosis

Microscopically, both infiltrative and hy-perplastic changes are visible. Campylobac-ter sp. have been isolated from affected ferrets.   H&E stain.

Transmissible Colonic Hyperplasia of Mice (TCHM)

Citrobacter freundii is the etiologic agent for this murine enterocolonic infection. It causes marked hyperplasia of the mucosal epithelial cells and minimal inflammation.

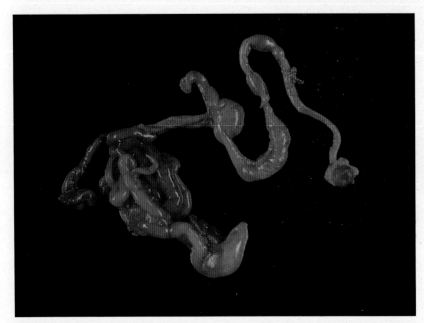

Plates 411,412   TCHM

Thickening of the colon wall is the characteristic feature of this disease. Normal colon and cecum are included for comparison.

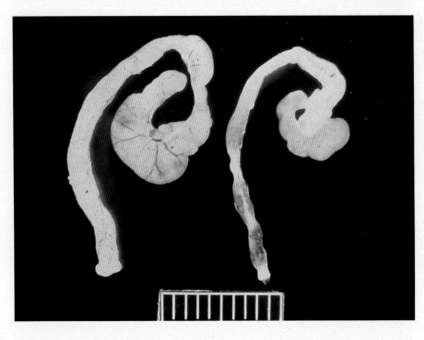

Plate 412   TCHM

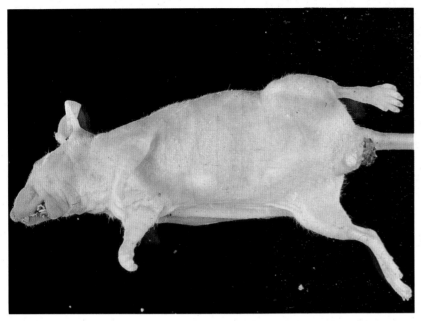

Plate 413   TCHM

In addition to diarrhea, mice with TCHM frequently develop anal prolapse due to straining.

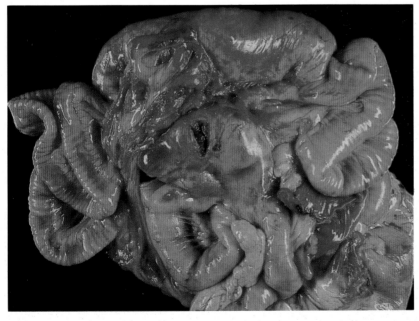

Plates 414,415   Canine Pythiosis

As elsewhere in the alimentary tract, the intestinal tract can be involved to manifest a severe necrotizing pyogranulomatous inflammation.

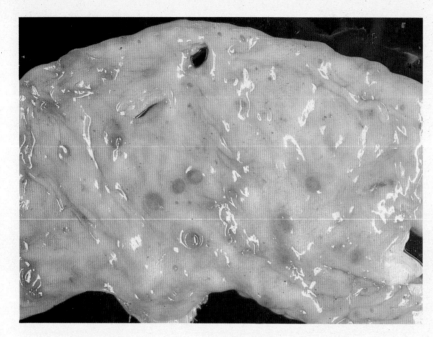

Plate 415   Canine Pythiosis

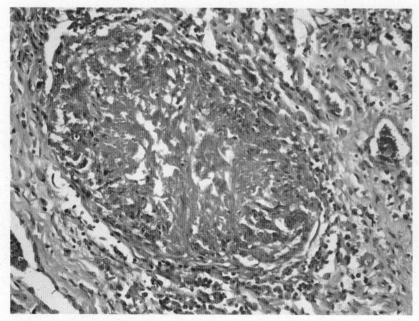

Plate 416   Canine Pythiosis
Microscopically, discrete confluent granulo
mas are hallmark lesions for infection
with Pythium.

VII. Intestinal Parasites

The contribution of endoparasites to disease depends on the number of worms present, on the degree of injury that they inflict, on the host tissue and on the syndrome that can be associated with the presence of worms such as diarrhea, wasting, hypoproteinemia and anemia. The following Plates are representations of nematodal, cestodal, trematodal and protozoal infestations.

Hookworms

Members of the genus Ancylostoma usually inhabit the small intestine where they loosely attach to the mucosal surface. Adults are bloodsuckers that can cause severe anemia and hypoproteinemia in heavy infestations. Blood is also directly lost into the intestinal tract of hookworm-infestated animals.

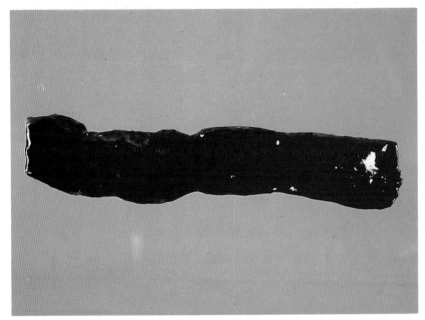

Plate 417   Canine Hookworms

Blood loss into intestinal tract is severe.

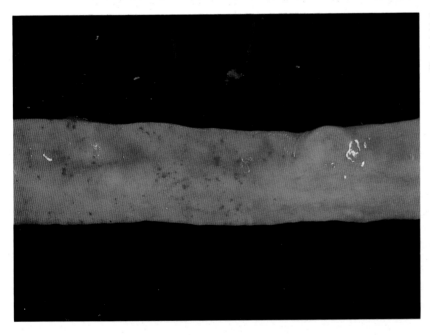

Plate 418   Canine Hookworms

Punctate red foci indicate attachment sites on mucosa.

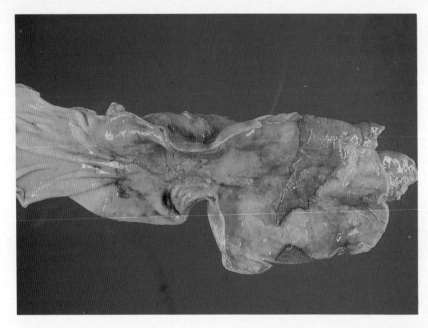

Plate 419   Canine Hookworm

Chronic antigen stimulation by worms is reflected by hyperplastic lymphoid nodules.

Trichuris

These are thin worms that inhabit the cecum or colon of domestic animals.   The life cycle is direct. Heavy infestation is associated with diarrhea or dysentery.

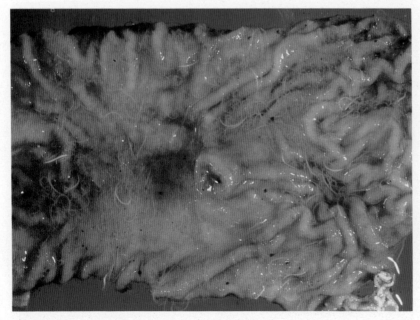

Plate 420   Porcine Trichuriasis

Note the mucus contents in cecum.

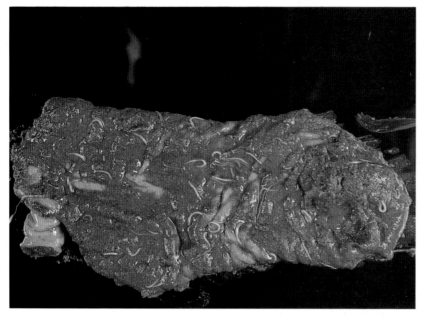

Plate 421   Caprine Trichuriasis

Thin worms are interspersed between larger ingesta particles.

Oesophagostomum

Members of the genus affect cattle, sheep and swine. The worms characteristically form discrete, transmural nodules in the small and large intestine. These nodules have a tendency to mineralize. Severe infestation can cause hypoproteinemia, wasting and death.

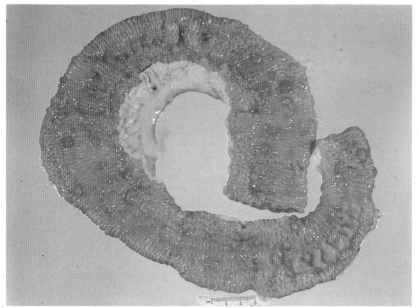

Plate 422   Bovine Oesophagostomiasis

Many glistening nodules bulge the mucosa.

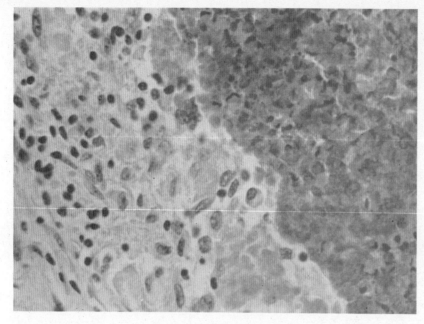

Plate 423   Bovine Oesophagostomiasis

Microscopically, the nematode elicits a foreign-body inflammatory response with macrophages, giant cells and inspissated eosinophils.

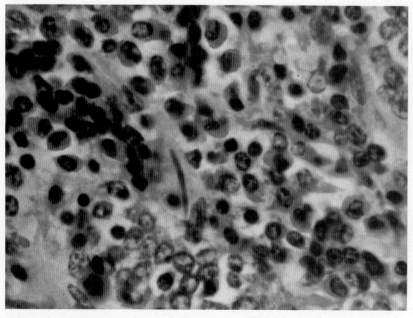

Plate 424   Bovine Oesophagostomiasis

Florid microscopic changes are characterized by a predominantly eosinophilic infiltrate in the lamina propria and submucosa.

Strongyloides

The diagnosis of Strongyloides infestation usually is made on flotation or microscopically. Adult worms are difficult to identify with the naked eye. In most animal species, the cranial small intestine is affected.

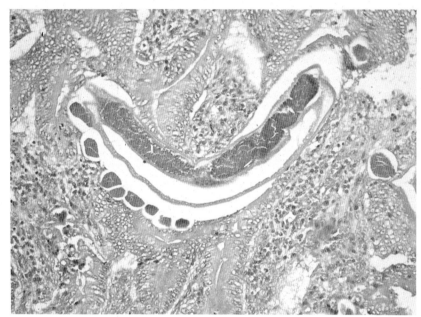

Plate 425 Feline Strongyloidosis

In cats, Strongyloides tumefaciens affects the colon by forming submucosal nodules as response. The plate shows the presence of colonic glands in the submucosa and larval cross-sections.

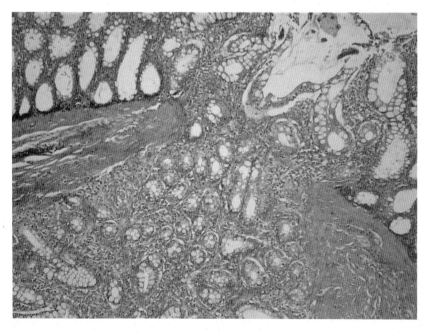

Plate 426 Feline Strongyloidosis

There is marked hyperplasia of cryptal epithelium around nematode larvae and ova.

Equine Strongylosis

Strongylinae are subdivided into large and small strongyles. While adults cause little tissue damage, the larvae of the large strongyles have a tendency to migrate through the abdominal cavity of the horse to induce disease. Small strongyles are known as Cyathostominae. The adult forms are harmless to the host, while the larvae migrate locally through the mucosa and submucosa of the large colon.

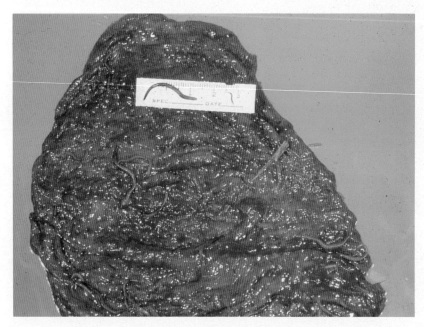

Plate 427   Strongylosis
Large and small strongyles attach to the mucosal surface of the colon.

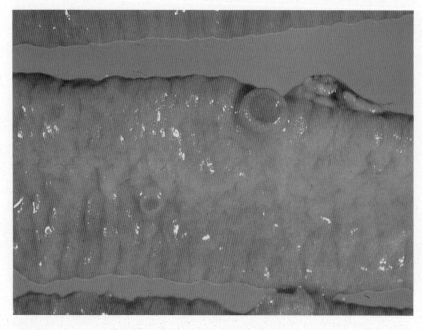

Plate 428   Strongylosis
Attachment sites of small strongyles (Cyathostominae)

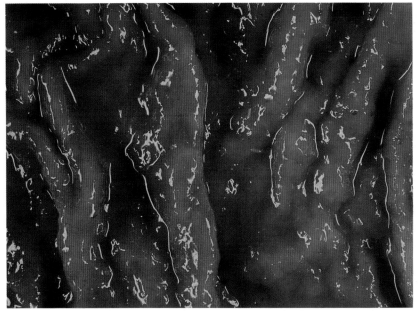

Plate 429   Strongylosis

Adults of Cyathostominae sp. are barely visible.

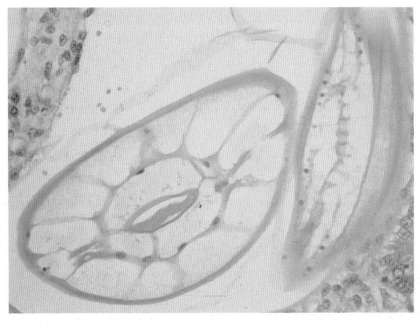

Plate 430   Strongylosis

Cross-section through adult of small strongylus. H&E stain.

Ascariasis

Ascarids are important endoparasites of swine, horses and carnivores. Larval migration through various internal organs is common and tissue destruction may be significant in some animal species. The life cycle is direct.

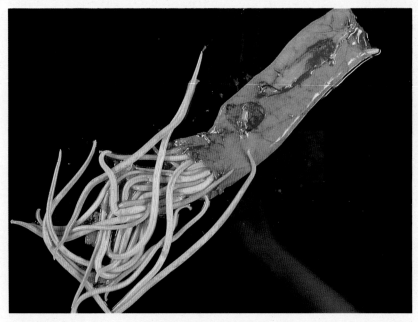

Plates 431,432 Parascaris Equorum

The nematodes have a tendency to crowd the small intestine in young untreated horses. Perforation may result from heavy parasite burden.

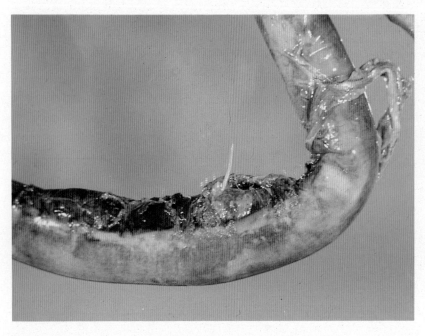

Plate 432 Parascaris Equorum

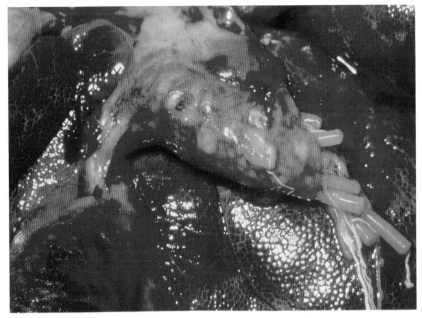

Plates 433,434 Ascaris Suum

The adult pig ascarid can be quite long. Heavy infestation of the bile duct may cause obstructive icterus.

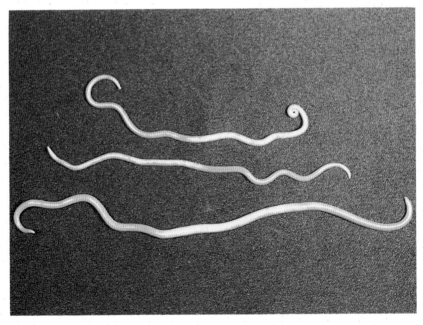

Plate 434   Ascaris Suum

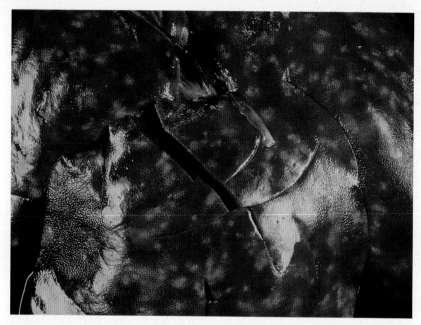

Plate 435   Ascaris Suum
Larval migration induces lesions in the liver and lung. In the liver, migration tracts heal by fibrosis to induce "milk spots".

Cestodiasis

Generally, adult tapeworms are of less pathogenicity than nematodes in their habitat. Cestodes are found in ruminants, carnivores and horses.

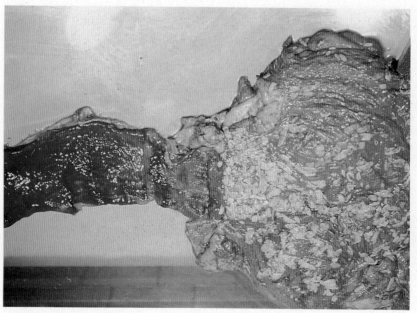

Plate 436   Equine Cestodes
Anoplocephala perfoliata colonizes the proximal cecum in horses. Heavy infestation causes an occasional ileo-cecal orifice obstruction or ileo-cecal intussusception. Erosive, fibrinous typhlitis also occurs from attachment of the worms.

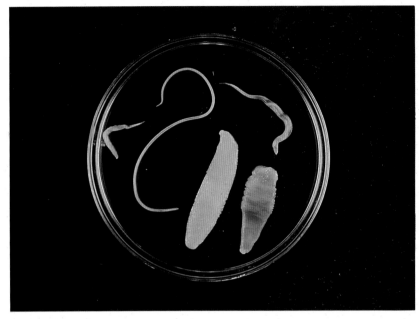

Plate 437   Equine Parasites

The dish contains small and large strongyles together with cestodes and Sertaria sp.

Intestinal Schistosomiasis

The presence of a multifocal granulomatous enteritis associated with wasting and the identification of parasites within mesenteric veins suggest infestation with Schistosoma sp. in ruminants and Heterobilharzia sp. in dogs.   Occasionally, horses in the southeast of the US are found to be infestated with   schistosomes.

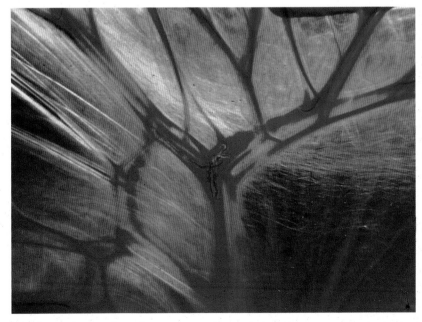

Plate 438   Bovine Schistosomiasis

Adult worms are visible in stretched mesenteric vessels.

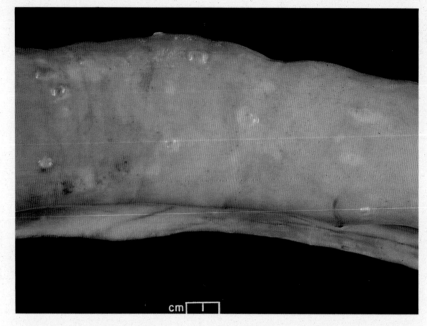

Plate 439   Equine Schistosomiasis

Several raised nodules occupy the serosa of the small intestine of a horse with severe weight loss and signs of chronic liver failure.

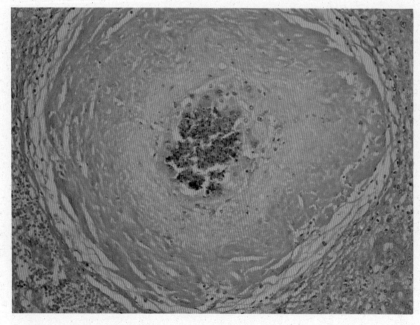

Plates 440,441   Equine Schistosomiasis

Histologically, the nodules are composed of a fibrous granuloma with central necrosis and an occasional ovum that has a pigmented wall typical of fluke eggs. H&E stain.

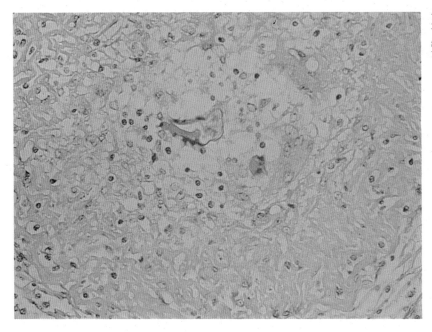

Plate 441   Equine Schistosomia-sis

Coccidiosis

Coccidia are intracellular parasites with a typical specificity towards host, organ and tissue. They are protozoa belonging to the phylum Apicomplexa. The number of sporocysts and sporozoites is used as characteristic to differentiate various genera of coccidia. Lesions characteristic of coccidiosis are located at the site of parasitism. The life cycle is direct. There are asexual and sexual stages.

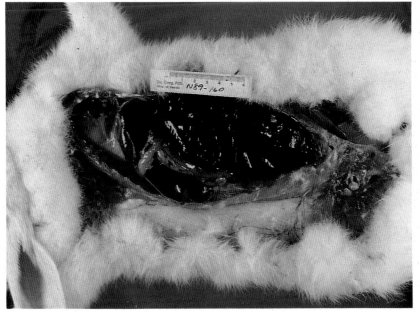

Plate 442   Rabbit Coccidiosis

Grossly, the presence of intestinal hemorrhage suggests necrosis and vascular insult.

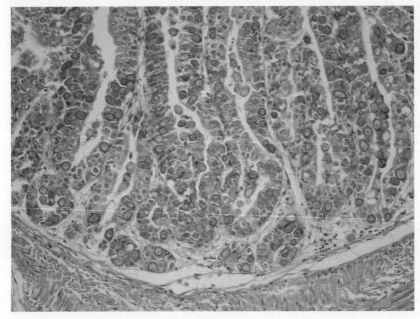

Plate 443   Rabbit Coccidiosis
Microscopically, the intestinal epithelium is studded with macrogametes of Eimeria sp. H&E stan.

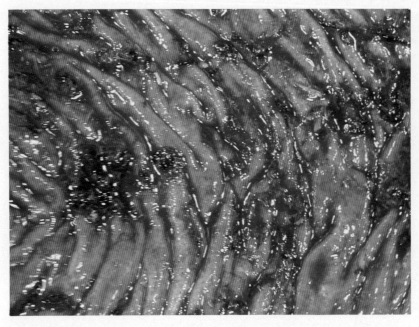

Plate 444   Bovine Coccidiosis
Fibrino-hemorrhagic typhlocolitis in seven-month old bovine infected with Eimeria sp.

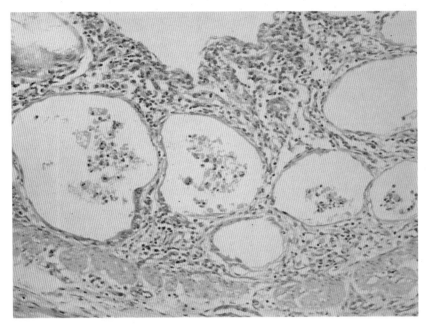

Plate 445   Bovine Coccidiosis

Microscopically, the glandular epithelium of the colon is attenuated. A few metaplastic epithelial lining cells, neutrophils and occasional oocysts are entrapped in distended glands.   H&E stain.

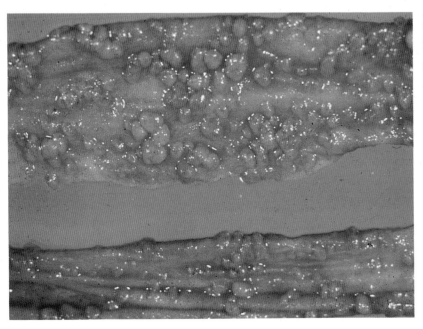

Plate 446   Caprine Coccidiosis

Goat coccidiosis is encountered in young animals.   Discrete nodular elevations are visible on the mucosal surface.

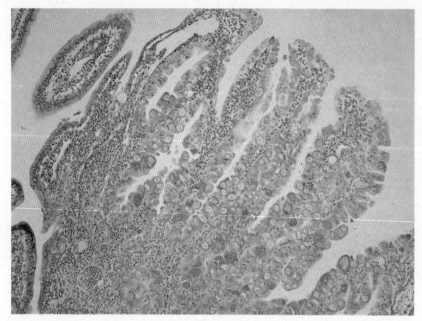

Plate 447   Caprine Coccidiosis
The nodules are the result of hypertrophy of the villus epithelium where virtually every epithelial cell is infected by mainly gametocytic stages of coccidia, in this case Eimeria arloingi. H&E stain.

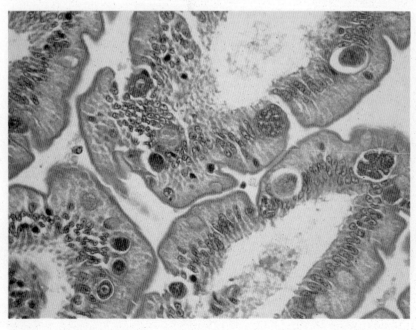

Plate 448   Feline Coccidiosis
Intestine of cat with multinucleate basophilic microgametes and uninucleate eosinophilic macrogametes present in the epithelial cells. H&E stain.

Cryptosporidiosis

Cryptosporidium sp. are intracellular, coccidian parasites that have been found to colonize the small and large intestines of calves, horses, rabbits, monkeys, cats, dogs, poultry and man. In immunocompetent hosts, a self-limiting diarrhea develops; in immunodeficient hosts, infection may result in a life-threatening condition. The protozoan has an asexual and sexual life cycle.

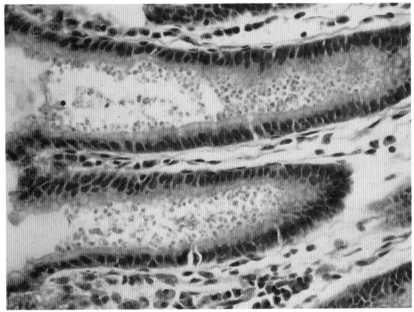

Plates 449,450 Cryptosporidiosis

Coccoid, round organisms are located on the surface of the abomasum and in the brush border of the jejunum of a calf. H&E stain.

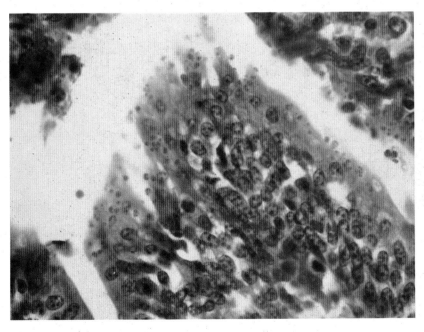

Plate 450 Cryptosporidiosis

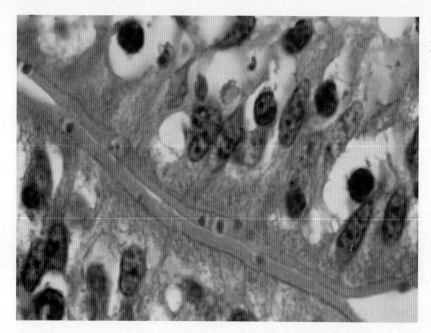

Plate 451 Cryptosporidiosis
Piglet infected with Cryptosporidium sp.

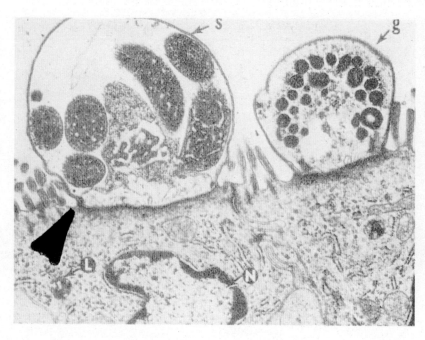

Plate 452 Cryptosporidiosis
Electronmicroscopically, it becomes evident that Cryptosporidium occupies the microvillus border of enterocytes and that it is partially surrounded by portions of the cell membrane (arrow). Merozoites are visible in the center of a meront.

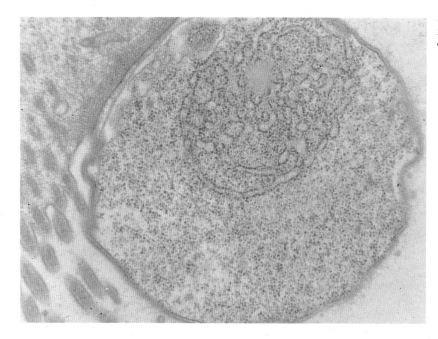

Plate 453   Cryptosporidiosis

Transmission electron micrograph.

Giardiasis

The disease is caused by a flagellated protozoan. Giardia lamblia. Its disk attaches to the epithelial surface of the intestinal tract. The agent has been reported to interfere with sugar absorption and to increase intestinal osmosis with watery diarrhea as the net result. Giardia exists in two phases:trophozoite and cyst. Each cyst contains two trophozoites.   Animals ingest the cysts from contaminated water. Inside the stomach, trophozoites are released to attach to the epithelium of the small intestine.   The organism has two equal-sized nuclei resembling "eyes".

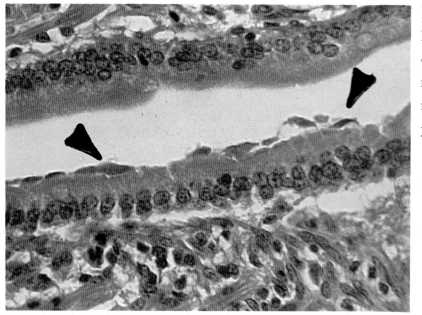

Plates 454,455   Giardiasis

Microscopically, Giardia can be easily overlooked as it takes up ring- or banana- shaped forms mimicking inspissated mucin (arrow) as in this duodenum of a young dog. H&E stain.

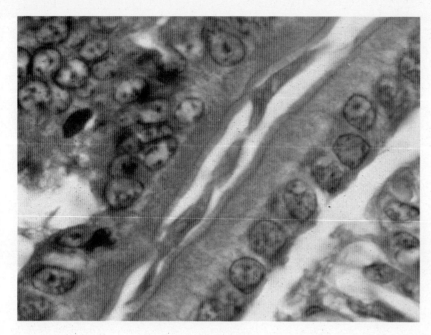

Plate 455   Giardiasis

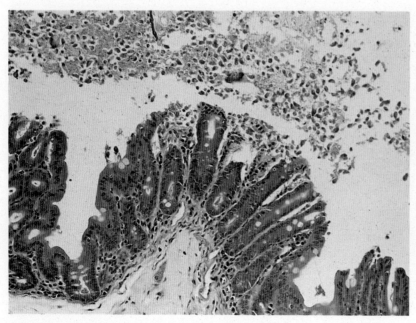

Plates 456,457 Porcine Tri-chomoniasis

Chronic diarrhea in conjunction with diar-rhea may in some instances be associated with infection by the flagellate Tritri-chomonas in pigs, horses and cattle. H&E stain.

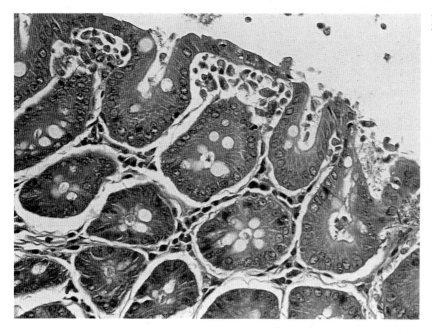

Plate 457 Trichomoniasis

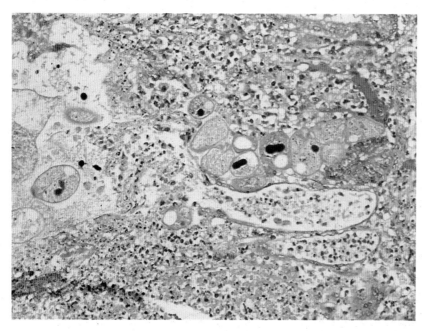

Plate 458 Balantidium Coli

The large, oval, ciliated protozoan can be found in the colon of pigs, humans, non-human primates and occasionally in horses and dogs. Usually a commensal, it can become an opportunistic pathogen once certain preceding colonic events develop. Under these circumstances, the protozoan is visible in the vicinity of necrotic or ulcerative lesions and is easily recognizable by its size and large, kidney-shaped nucleus as is illustrated in this pig with a necrotizing colitis.

VIII. Intestinal Neoplasms

According to the cell of origin, tumors are of either epithelial or mesenchymal lineage. Occasional intestinal neoplasms are derived from neuroendocrine cells of the APUD system. Epithelial tumors are either polyps, adenomas or carcinomas. They usually occur in the duodenal or colon-rectal segments of the intestinal tract. Mesenchymal neoplasms arise mainly from smooth muscle cells of the tunica muscularis to develop leiomyomas or leiomyosarcomas. The majority of mesenchymal tumors in animals are lymphosarcomas. Most intestinal neoplasms are encountered in dogs and cats. Sporadic cases have been reported in sheep, cattle and horses.

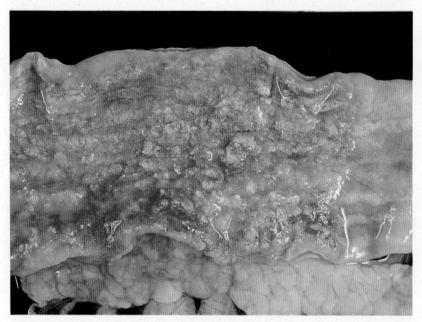

Plate 459 Duodenal Carcinoma
An elevated, plaque-like intraluminal mass is occupying the anterior duodenum of a dog.

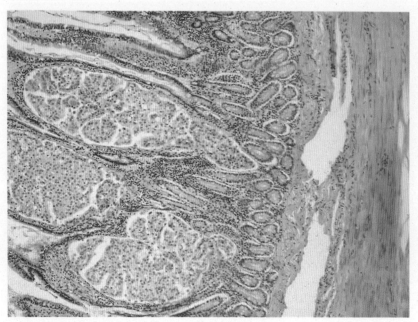

Plate 460 Duodenal Carcinoma
Sheets and ribbons of neoplastic epithelial cells have invaded the lamina propria and have distended duodenal villi. H&E stain.

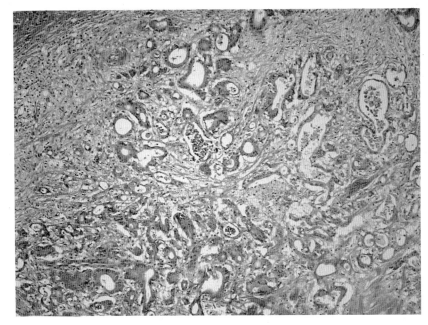

Plate 461 Duodenal Carcinoma

Individual neoplastic cells and neoplastic acinar formations are present in the sub-mucosa. H&E stain.

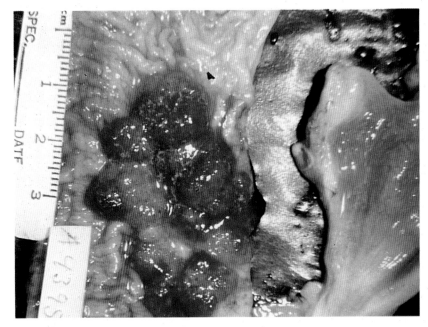

Plate 462 Colorectal Polyp

A four-year old dog with unresponsive diarrhea and dyschezia had several fleshy sessile nodules of several centimeters in the mucosa at the colorectal junction.

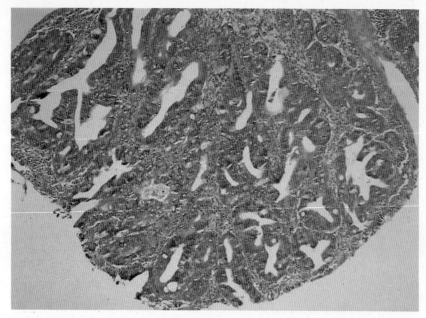

Plate 463   Colorectal Polyp

Microscopically, the growth is characterized by branching, papillary projections of differentiated columnar epithelial cells that project into the intestinal lumen. Rectal polyps have to be differentiated from polypoid adenomas and carcinomas. H&E stain.

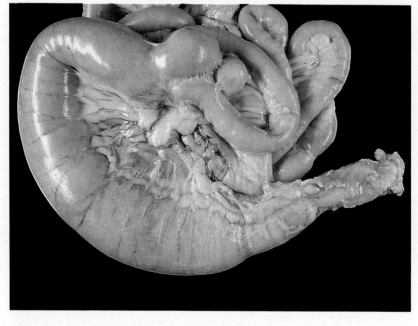

Plates 464,465 Colonic Adenocarcinoma

An annular constriction with thickening of the wall affects the terminal colon of a dog.

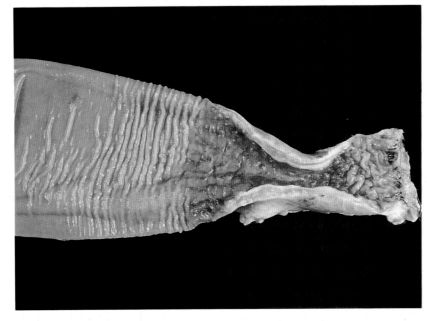

Plate 465 Colonic Adenocarcinoma

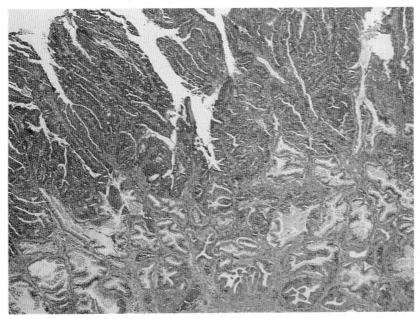

Plates 466,467 Colonic Adenocarcinoma

Microscopically, the tumor has polypoid features on the mucosal surface with lumenal papillary projections, whereas individual neoplastic cells have invaded the lamina propria, submucosa and muscularis and, via lymphatics, mesenteric lymph nodes. H&E stain.

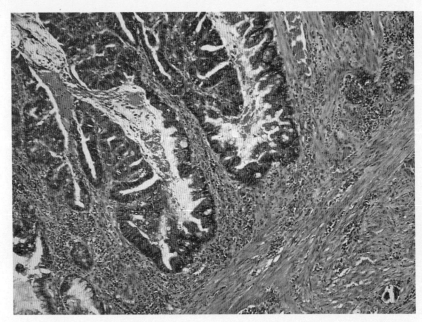

Plate 467 Colonic Adenocarcinoma

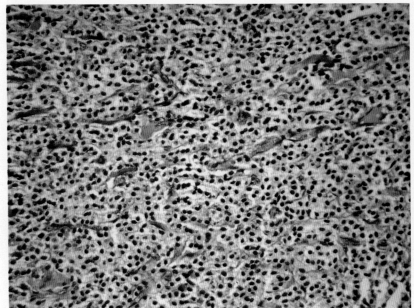

Plate 468 Intestinal Carcinoid

Carcinoids have an endocrine appearance at the microscopic level. The neoplastic cells may secrete biogenic amines which stain positively with argentaffinic and argyrophilic stains, but do not stain metachromatically or with PAS stains. This tumor occurred in a cat. H&E stain.

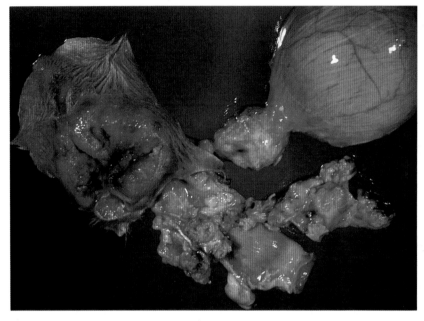

Plate 469   Perianal Gland Tumors

Tumors located in the canine perineum may originate from various glandular structures characteristic for the region, in particular from perianal glands, anal sac and anal sac glands. The vast majority arise from perianal (hepatoid) glands and exhibit benign features. The tumors occur predominantly in male dogs; castration is recommended as preventive therapy following surgical excision. Perianal tumors are manifested clinically as growths bulging from the anus and into the surrounding perirectal soft tissue.

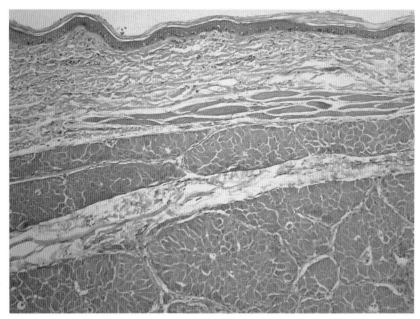

Plate 470   Perianal Gland Adenoma

Histologically, most perianal tumors are benign and exhibit a differentiated growth pattern of lobules of large, polyhedral cells with abundant eosinophilic cytoplasm. The histologic aspects of the tumor cells correspond well with the features of normal perianal glands close by. H&E stain.

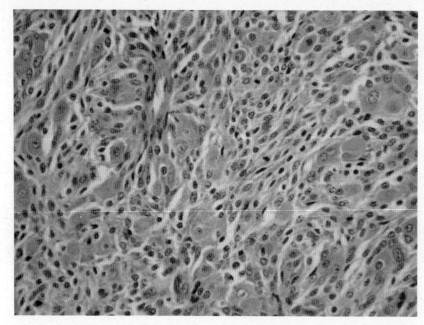

Plate 471　Perianal Gland Carcinoma

Perianal gland carcinomas are rare and lack perianal gland differentiation. Instead, groups of reserve cells create a picture of hypercellularity. Mitotic figures and lymphatic invasion are additional features of malignancy. H&E stain.

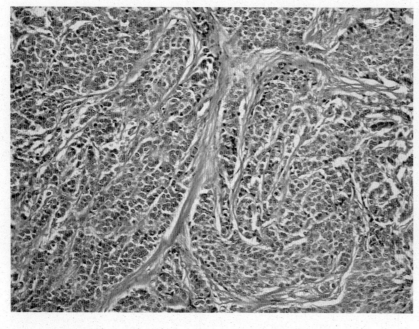

Plates 472,473　Adenocarcinoma of Canine Anal Sac Glands

These predominantly malignant tumors are comprised of solid groups of neoplastic cells separated by fine connective tissue strands that contain capillaries. The tumor cells are fairly small with nuclear hyperchromasia. Occasional rosettes or tubular patterns may be present. Hypercalcemia has been reported in 90% of dogs developing this particular type of perineal neoplasm. Other clinical signs may include polyuria/ polydipsia, muscular weakness, lethargy, anorexia and vomiting. H&E stain.

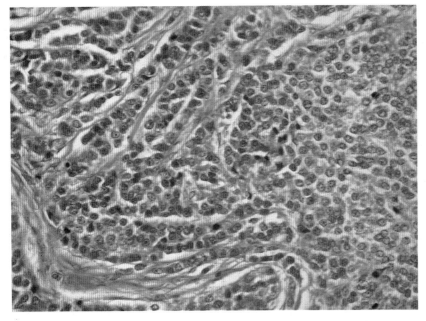

Plate 473 Adenocarcinoma of Canine Anal Sac Glands

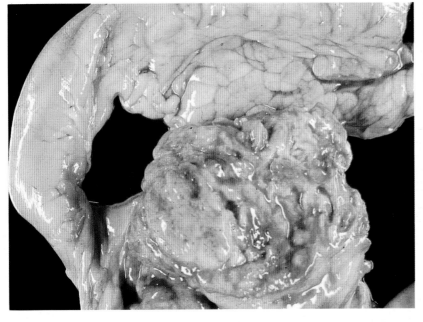

Plate 474 Jejunal Leiomyosarcoma

A nodular, ulcerative growth in an older dog was the cause of partial obstruction.

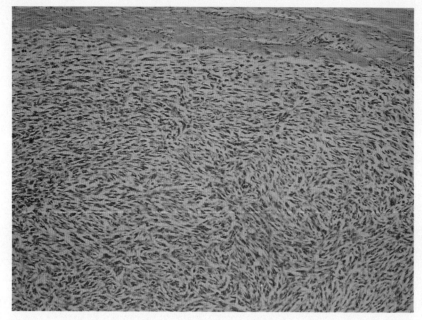

Plate 475   Jejunal Leiomyosarcoma

Microscopically, the neoplasm is comprised of smooth muscle cells. H&E stain.

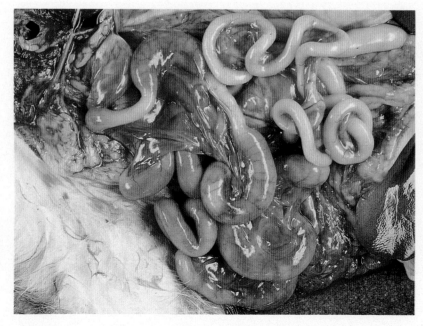

Plate 476   Intestinal Lymphosarcoma

Lymphosarcomas are the most common types of intestinal neoplasms in cats. The tumor may be solitary, or multiple as in this feline case.

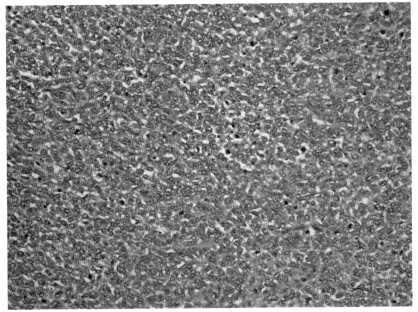

Plate 477 Intestinal Lymphosarcoma

The histologic appearance is similar to lymphosarcomas in other sites. H&E stain.

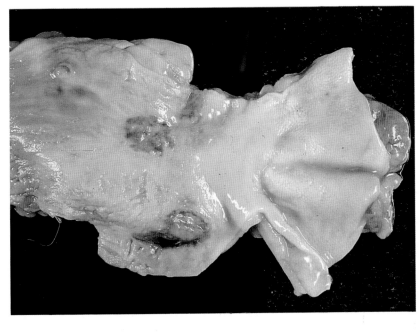

Plate 478   Intestinal Mast Cell Tumor

Mast   cell tumors usually arise in the small intestine. They are more frequent in cats than in dogs, but overall are rare tumors. Affected areas in the gut are thickened, velvety, raised and ulcerated as seen in the duodenum of a dog.

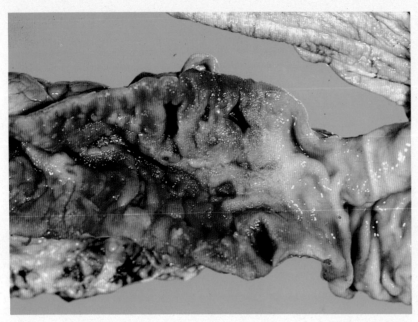

Plate 479 Duodenal Ulcers

In the dog, cutaneous mast cell tumors may cause ulcers in the duodenum (or stomach) due to excessive histamine production.

IX. Miscellaneous

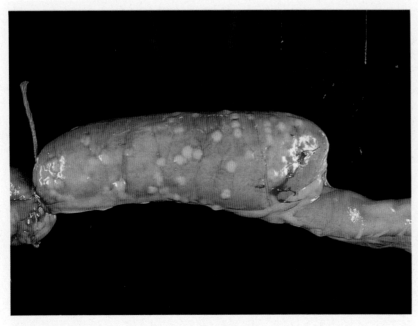

Plate 480 Lymphoid Hyperplasia

Prominent lymphoid follicles in the cecum of a young dog should not be confused with true pathologic lesions such as necrosis, ulcers, inflammation. The follicles develop in response to antigen stimulation.

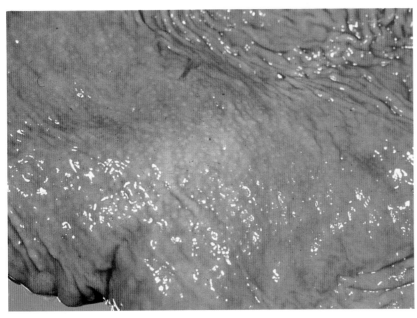

Plate 481 Lymphoid Hyperplasia

Stimulated lymphoid follicles are visible as small white granules within the mucosa of the colon of a young horse.

Intestinal Lymphangiectasia

Primary lymphangiectasia has been reported in puppies as congenital malformation of intestinal or mesenteric lymphatic vessels. (Segmental aplasia resulting in failure of continuity).

Secondary forms are the result of lymphangitis, lymphatic thrombosis or stricture of lymphatics. Both types are clinically associated with protein-losing enteropathy and malabsorption.

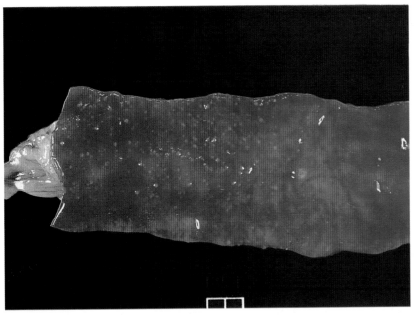

Plate 482 Lymphangiectasia

Distended lymphatics are grossly visible as small white spots in the reddened mucosa. Post-prandial distention of lymphatics occurs after the consumption of a fat-rich diet (physiologic lymphangiectasia).

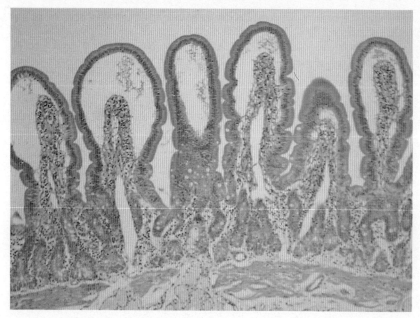

Plates 483,484 Lymphangiectasia

Dilated lacteals in the tips of villi are the result of lymph stasis from obstruction of intestinal or mesenteric lymphatics. The villi are markedly widened, and the lamina propria is spongy. H&E stain.

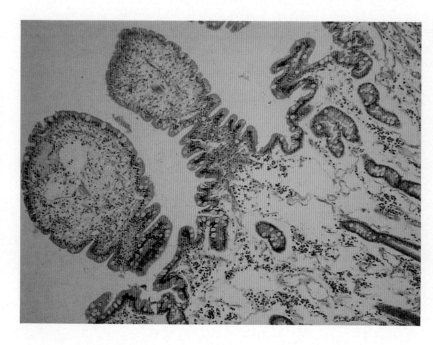

Plate 484　Lymphangiectasia

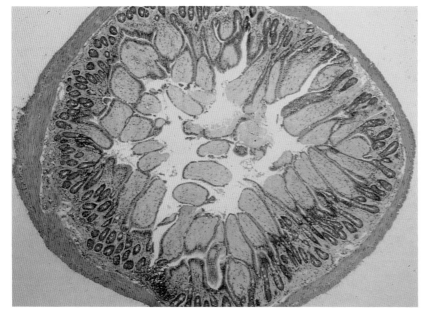

Plate 485   Intestinal Amyloidosis

The lamina propria of this mouse's ileum is distended with amorphous, eosinophilic material identified as amyloid. H&E stain.

Intestinal Lipofuscinosis ("Brown Gut Disease")

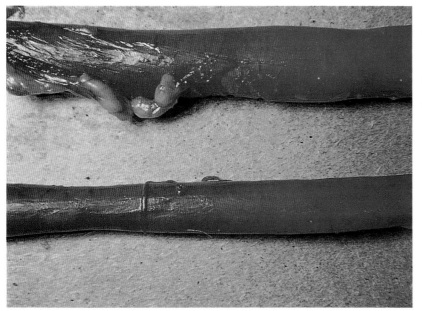

Plate 486   Lipofuscinosis

This incidental finding in dogs is a lesion of the past. The brown discoloration is thought to be due to vitamin E deficiency in the diet.

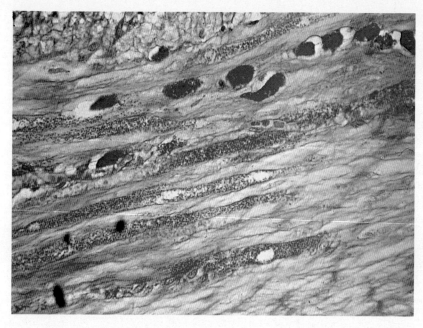

Plate 487　Lipofuscinosis
Histologically, PAS- positive pigment granules are deposited in the cytoplasm of the smooth muscle cells of the tunica muscularis. The granules also are acid-fast positive and represent lipofuscin pigment. PAS stain.

Equine Hemomelasma Ilei
Focal, subserosal, red-to-black patches in the serosa represent hemorrhagic infarcts postulated to be the result of aberrantly migrating larvae of Strongylus sp. These are incidental findings at necropsy.

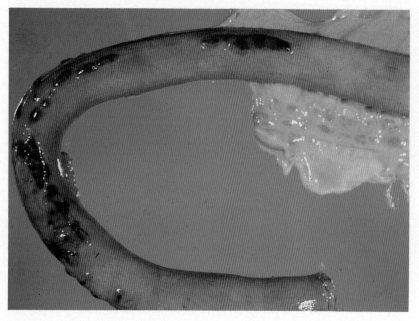

Plates 488,489　H. Ilei
Gross appearance of hemomelasma ilei. The typical location is opposite the mesenteric attachment to the gut.

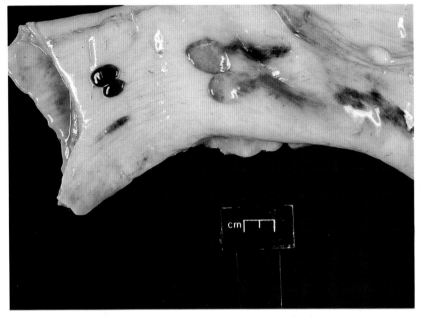

Plate 489   H. Ilei

Plate 490   H. Ilei

Microscopically, hemosiderin-laden macrophages are indicative of hemorrhagic suffusion into the subserosal tissue. Organization of hemorrhage is further indicated by the presence of angioblasts, capillaries and fibroblasts. H&E stain.

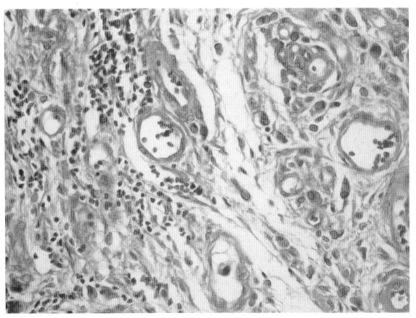

Megacolon

This disorder occurs as congenital or acquired form.If congenital, it is associated with aganglionosis (hypoganglionosis) of the colon.

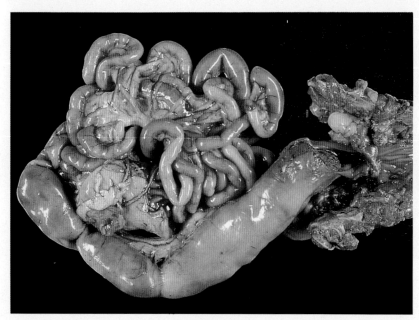

Plate 491 Megacolon

Acquired forms of megacolon occur after traumas to the pelvis or terminal spinal cord nerves as happened to this cat.

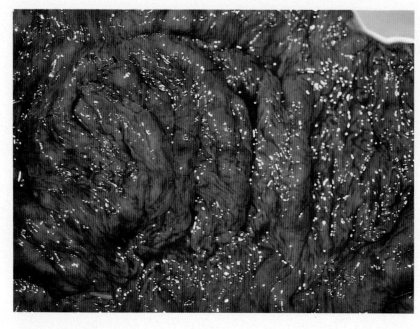

Plate 492 Uremic Colitis

The mucosal surface of the colon shows both white plaques and diffuse reddening in a horse with chronic renal failure.

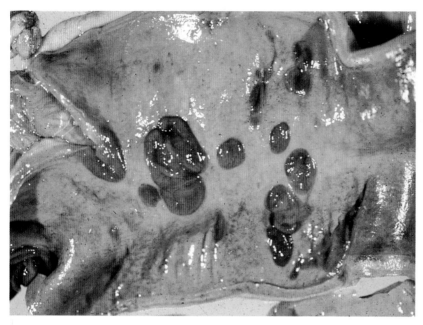

Plate 493 Right Dorsal Colitis

Ulcerative lesions uniquely localized in the right dorsal colon have been reported in horses treated with nonsteroidal anti-inflammatory drugs. Typically, large areas of the mucosa of the right dorsal colon have disappeared with only a few mucosal remnants left. It is not known why the lesions are localized preferentially in the right dorsal colon.

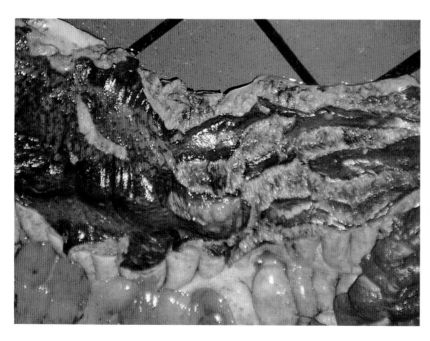

Plate 494 Equine Salmonellosis

The entity of right dorsal ulcerative colitis has to be differentiated from equine salmonellosis.

Equine Duodenitis-Proximal Jejunitis (EDPJ)

This newer equine disorder also is known as anterior enteritis. Colic, copious gastric reflux and the development of laminitis are major clinical features. The cause remains unknown, but Clostridium organisms are suspected. Toxicosis is ruled out due to the sporadic nature of the disease.

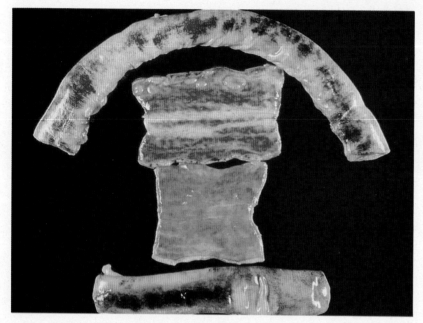

Plates 495–497 EDPJ

The gross changes in the affected intestine vary from a few serosal petechiae to severe transmural hemorrhages and yellow discolorations.

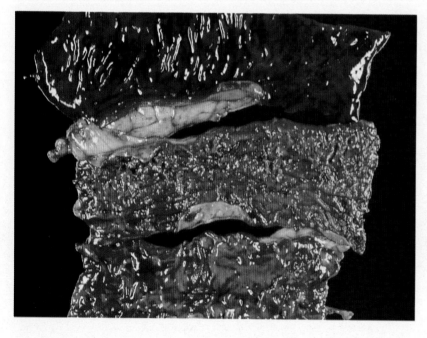

Plate 496 EDPJ

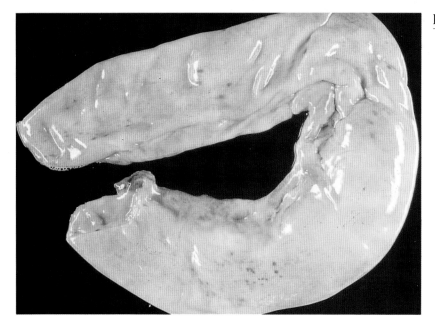

Plate 497 EDPJ

Equine Granulomatous Enteritis (EGE)

Equine granulomatous enteritis and equine chronic eosinophilic enteritis are two distinct chronic intestinal entities that mimic intestinal mycobacteriosis. The disorders have been reported from Sweden, Australia and North America. Affected horses were mostly young standardbreds. The etiology for both equine granulomatous enteritis and equine chronic eosinophilic enteritis remains obscure. No specific agent could be identified.

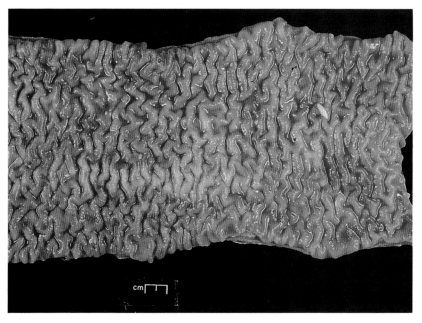

Plate 498 EGE

Typical gross changes are uniformly thick and prominent intestinal mucosal folds of the caudal small intestine. Mesenteric lymph nodes are enlarged.

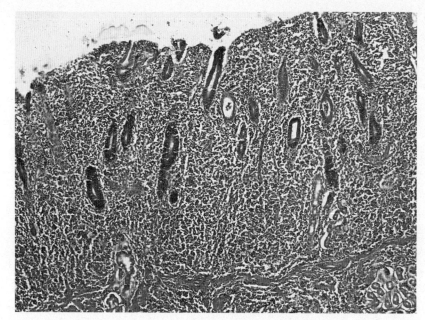

Plates 499,500   EGE

Lymphocytes, macrophages and epithelioid cells have diffusely accumulated in the lamina propria causing villous atrophy and obliteration.   Special stains or electronmicrography failed to identify a causative agent.   H&E stain.

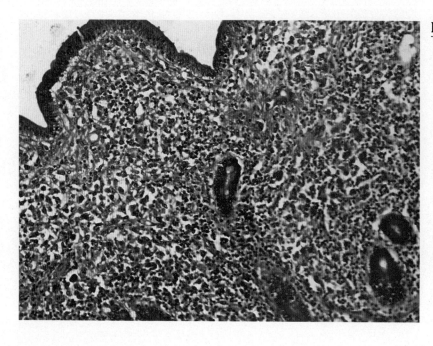

Plate 500   EGE

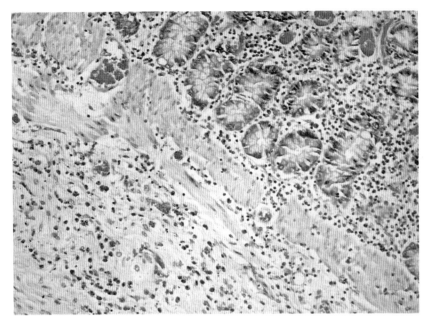

Plate 501 Equine Chronic Eosinophilic Enteritis (ECEE)

Eosinophils are the prominent inflammatory cell type in this entity. H&E stain.

Canine Lymphocytic-Plasmacytic Enteritis (LPE)

Chronic diarrhea. vomiting. weight loss and hypoproteinemia are non-specific clinical hallmarks of this canine disorder. A breed or sex predisposition has not been documented. The majority of affected dogs belong to the middle-age group. The principal cause remains unknown. Bacterial overgrowth. sprue-like enteropathy, hypersensitivity to intestinal nematodes or premalignant intestinal lymphosarcoma have been advanced as hypotheses. The diagnosis is made by endoscopic mucosal biopsy.

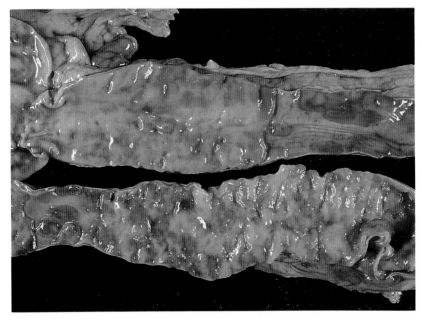

Plate 502 LPE

Rarely will the disease reveal itself as prominently at necropsy as seen in the duodenum and cranial jejunum of this dog with intestinal malabsorption.

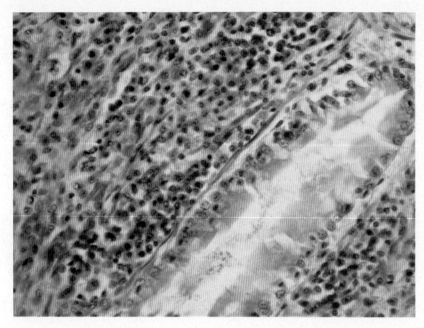

Plate 503 LPE

Microscopically. villi should be distinctly filled with lymphocytes and plasma cells to establish the diagnosis of LPE. Villus blunting. fusion and/or obliteration greatly substantiate the diagnosis. Caution is advised not to overdiagnose LPE since lymphocytes and plasma cells are normal intestinal resident cells.   H&E stain.

Chronic Canine Enteropathies

This diverse group of wasting diseases in dogs incorporates recognizable intestinal entities and non-recognizable chronic conditions. The principal microscopic changes are filling and obliteration of villi by inflammatory cells. interference with villus movement or absorption and obstruction of nutrient flux through blocked lacteals and capillaries.

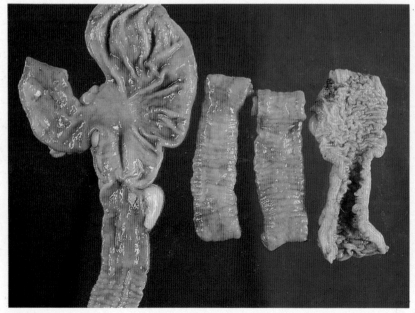

Plates 504,505 Chronic Canine Enteropathy

Grossly. most of the canine cases show marked mucosal thickening of a major segment of the cranial small intestinal tract. Caution should be exercised as to this being normal due to mucosal retraction.

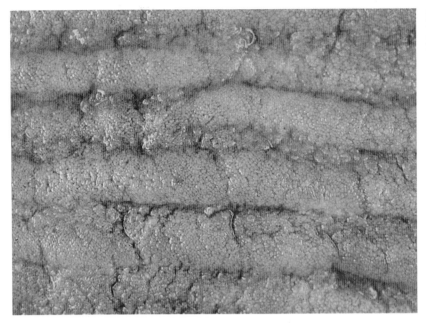

Plate 505 **Chronic Canine Enteropathy**

Literature

1. J.C. Baker: Bovine Viral Diarrhea: A Review. J. Am. Vet. Med. Assoc. 190:1449, 1987.

2. S.W. Barthold, G.L. Coleman, R.O. Jacoby, E.M. Livestone, A.M. Jonas: Transmissible Murine Colonic Hyperplasia. Vet. Path. 15:223, 1978.

3. R.M. Batt, E.J. Hall: Chronic Enteropathies in the Dog. J. Sm. Anim. Pract. 30:3, 1989.

4. J.L. Becht, S.D. Semrad: Gastrointestinal Diseases of Foals. Comp. Cont. Ed. 8:367, 1986.

5. J.E.C. Bellamy, S.D. Acres: Enterotoxigenic Colibacillosis in Colostrum-Fed Calves: Pathologic Changes. J. Am. Vet. Med. Assoc. 40:1391, 1979.

6. A. Berrocal, J.H. Vos, T. van den Ingh et al.: Canine Perineal Tumors. J. Vet. Med. A 36:739, 1989.

7. C.D. Buergelt, C. Hall, K. McEnty, J.R. Duncan: Pathological Evaluation of Paratuberculosis in Naturally Infected Cattle. Vet. Path. 15:196, 1978.

8. C.D. Buergelt, S.L. Green, I.G. Mayhew et al: Avian Mycobacteriosis in Three Horses. Cornell Vet. 78: 365, 1988.

9. D.O. Cordes, B.D. Pery, Y. Rikilisa, W.R. Chickening: Enterocolitis Caused by Ehrlichia sp. in the Horse (Potomac Horse Fever). Vet. Path. 23:471, 1986.

10. W.L. Current: Cryptosporidiosis. J. Am. Vet. Med. Assoc. 12:1334, 1985.

11. J.O. Gebbers, J.A. Laissue: Immunologic Structures and Functions of the Gut. Schw. Arch. Tierhlk. 131: 221, 1989.

12. J.T. Harkin, R.T. Jones, J.C. Gillick: Rectal Strictures in Pigs. Austr. Vet. J. 59:56, 1982.

13. P.J.K. Durham, L.E. Hassard, G.R. Norman et al: Viruses and Virus-like Particles Detected During Examination of Feces from Calves and Piglets with Diarrhea. Can. Vet. J. 30:876, 1989.

14. G. Jacobs, L. Collins-Kelly, M. Lappin et al: Lymphocytic-Plasmacytic Enteritis in 24 Dogs. J. Vet. Int. Med. 4:45, 1990.

15. R.O. Jacoby: Transmissible Ileal Hyperplasia of Hamsters. Am. J. Path. 91:433, 1978.

16. G.St. Jean, Y. Couture, P. Dubrevil et al: Diagnosis of Giardia Infection in 14 Calves. J. Am. Vet. Med. Assoc. 191:831, 1987.

17. E. A. Johnson, R.O. Jacoby: Transmissible Ileal Hyperplasia of Hamsters. Am. J. Path. 91:451, 1978.

18. J.A. Johnson, J.F. Rescott, R.J.F. Marklan: The Pathology of Experimental C. Equi Infection in Foals Following Intragastric Challenge. Vet. Path. 20:450, 1983.

19. L.F. Karcher, St.G. Dill, W.I. Anderson, J.M. King: Right Dorsal Colitis. J. Vet. Int. Med. 4:247, 1990.

20. T.H. Kent, H.W. Moon: The Comparative Pathogenesis of Some Enteric Diseases. Vet. Path. 10:414, 1973.

21. H.J. Kurtz, E.C. Short: Pathogenesis of Edema Disease in Swine: Pathologic Effects of Hemolysin, Autolysate and Endotoxin of E. Coli (0141). Am. J. Vet. Res. 37:15, 1976.

22. E.M. Liebler, J.F. Pohlenz, G.N. Woode: Gut-associated Lymphoid Tissue in the Large Intestine of

Calves. Vet. Path. 25:503 and 509, 1988.

23 . R. Lindberg: Pathology of Equine Granulomatous Enteritis. J. Comp. Path. 94:233, 1984.

24 . D.N. Love, R.J. Love: Pathology of Proliferative Haemorrhagic Enteropathy in Pigs. Vet. Path. 16:41, 1979.

25 . E.T. Lyons, J.A. Drudge, S.C. Tolliver: Review of Prevalence Surveys of Internal Parasites Recovered (1951-1990) from Horses at Necropsy in Kentucky. J. Eq. Vet. Sci 12:9, 1992.

26 . D.L. MacLeod, C.L. Gyles, P.P. Wilcock: Reproduction of Edema Disease of Swine with Purified Shiga-like Toxin-II Variant. Vet. Path. 28:66, 1991.

27 . S. McOrist, G.H. Lawson, A.C. Rowland, N. MacEntyre: Early Lesions of Proliferative Enteritis in Pigs and Hamsters . Vet. Path. 26:260, 1989.

28 . D.J. Meuten, G.V. Segre, C.C. Capen et al: Hypercalcemia in Dogs with Adenocarcinoma Derived from Apocrine Glands of the Anal Sac. Lab. Invest. 48:428, 1983.

29 . E. Momotani, D.Whipple, A.B. Tierman , N.F. Cheville: Role of M Cells and Macrophages in the Entrance of M. Paratuberculosis into Domes of Ileal Peyer's Patches in Calves. Vet. Path. 25:131, 1988.

30 . F. Moog: The Lining of the Small Intestine. Scient. Amer. 245:154, 1981.

31 . H.W. Moon: Mechanism in the Pathogenesis of Diarrhea: A Review. J. Am. Vet. Med. Assoc. 172:443, 1978.

32 . D.A. Moore, D.H. Zeman: Cryptosporidiosis in Neonatal Calves: 277 Cases (1986 -1987). Am J. Vet. Med. Assoc. 198:1969, 1991

33 . S.K. Nibbelink, M.J. Wannemuehler: Susceptibility of Inbred Mouse Strains to Infection with Serpulina (Treponema) hyodysenteriae. Infect. Immunity 59:3111, 1991.

34 . M. Reinacker: Feline Leukemia Virus-associated Enteritis: A Condition with Features of Feline Panleukopenia. Vet. Path. 24:1, 1987.

35 . M.C. Roberts: Malabsorption Syndromes in the Horse. Comp. Cont. Ed. 7:637, 1985.

36 . A.J. Roussel, R.H. Whitlock: Chronic Diarrhea in Cattle: Differential Diagnosis. Comp Cont. Ed. 12:423, 1990.

37 . R.J. Seiler: Colorectal Polyps of the Dog: A Clinicopathologic Study of 17 Cases. J. Am. Vet. Med. Assoc. 174:72, 1979.

38 . H.F. Stiles: Isolation of an Intracellular Bacterium from Hamsters (Mesocricetus auratus) with Proliferative Ileitis and Reproduction of the Disease with a Pure Culture. Infect. Immunity 59:3227, 1991.

39 . W.A.Walker, K.J. Isselbacher: Intestinal Antibodies. New Engl. J. Med. 297:767, 1977.

40 . G.E. Ward, N.L. Winkelman: Recognizing the Three Forms of Proliferative Enteritis in Swine. Vet. Med. 85:197, 1990.

41 . N.A. White, D.E. Tyler, R.B. Blackwell, D. Allen: Hemorrhagic, Fibrinonecrotic Duodenitis-Proximal Jejunitis in Horses: 20 Cases (1977-1984). J. Am. Vet. Med. Assoc. 190:311, 1987.

42 . B.P. Wilcock, H.J. Olander: Studies on the Pathogenesis of Swine Dysentery. I. Characterization of the

Lesions in Colons and Colonic Segments Inoculated with Pure Cultures of Colonic Contents Containing Treponema hyodysenteriae. Vet. Path. 16:450, 1979.

43 . I. van der Gaag, D. Tibboch: Intestinal Atresia and Stenosis in Animals: A Report of 34 Cases. Vet. Path. 17:565, 1980.

44 . H.J. vanKruiningen, C.B. Williams: Mucoid Enteritis of Rabbits. Vet. Path. 9:53, 1972.

45 . H.J. vanKruiningen, L.H. Kairallak, V.G. Sasserille et al: Calfhood Coronavirus Enterocolitis: A Clue to the Etiology of Winter Dysentery. Vet. Path. 24:564, 1987.

Chapter 5 Diseases of the Peritoneum

The normal peritoneum is a smooth, thin, glistening membrane that is kept moist by small amounts of fluid. Distinction should be made between antemortem and postmortem effusions and discolorations.

Hydroperitoneum refers to accumulation of excessive, watery, straw-colored fluid in the peritoneal cavity. This fluid is mostly non-inflammatory edema (ascites) as part of generalized edema, the result of chronic passive congestion or the sequela of implants of neoplasms onto the peritoneum.

Hemoperitoneum refers to accumulation of frank blood in the peritoneal cavity. This accumulation results from traumatic injuries to various visceral organs, from ruptured splenic hemangiomas or hemangiosarcomas or from toxicoses such as warfarin.

Uroperitoneum refers to the presence of urine in the abdomen resulting from a ruptured urinary bladder or ureter.

I. Degenerative Changes

Abdominal Herniations

Truo or false extra-abdominal herniations frequently occur in young animals. They may give rise to focal or generalized peritonitis or to intestinal incarcerations.

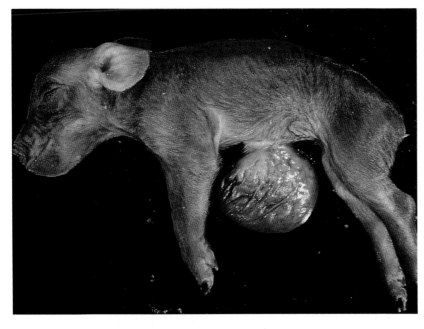

Plate 506   Hernia
Piglet with umbilical hernia.

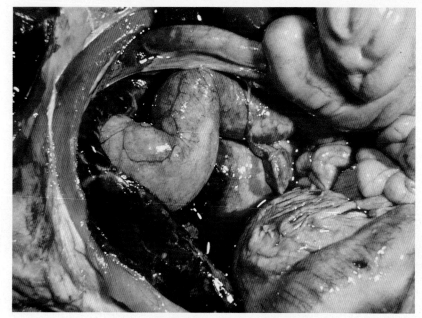

Plate 507   Hernia

An umbilical hernia leading to peritonitis in a calf.

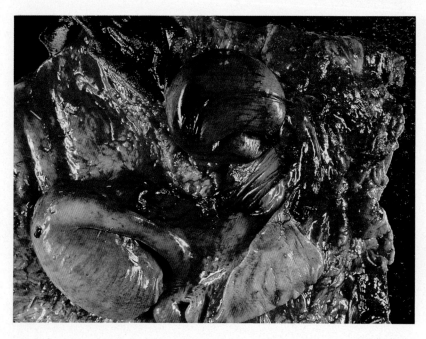

Plate 508   Hernia

An inguinal hernia in a horse resulting in intestinal strangulation.

Abdominal Fat Necrosis

Three types of necrosis of abdominal adipose tissue are recognized.

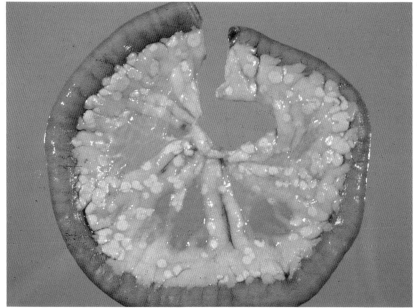

Plate 509   Peripancreatic Fat Necrosis

In pancreatic disease, enzymatic fat necrosis consistently occurs next to the pancreas and extends into the mesenteric tissue as in this cat.

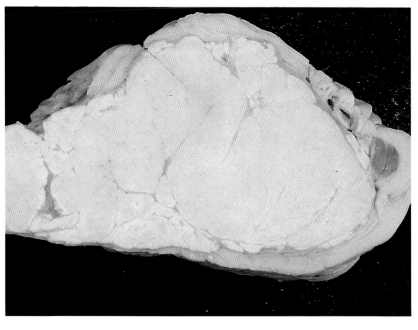

Plate 510   Focal Fat Necrosis

Focal, firm lobules of necrotic fat may randomly occur in the mesentery or omentum of obese sheep and horses. The necrosis is most likely ischemic in origin and is not accompanied by inflammation.

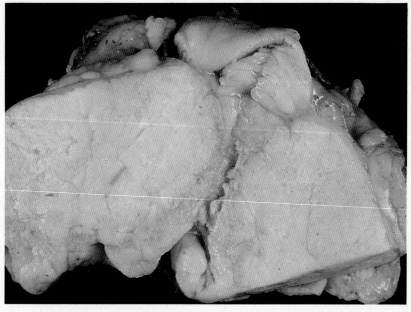

Plate 511   Extensive Fat Necro-sis

Abdominal fat necrosis of unclear (fescue grass?) origin occurs in cattle and is characterized by large masses of necrotic fat in the omentum, mesentery and retroperitoneal tissues. The masses on cut section are firm, dry or moist, and have a yellow color.

II.   Inflammations

Peritonitis is nearly always infectious. It is very common in large domestic animals. It may be serofibrinous, fibrinopurulent, purulent, granulomatous or fibrous, and whatever the type, it may be localized or generalized. The infection may subside, but adhesions and the formation of fibrous tissue may interfere with intestinal function. The majority of cases of peritonitis are caused by bacteria and their toxins. Feline infectious peritonitis is an example of a disease caused by a virus. The principal routes by which infections spread throughout the peritoneal cavity are:

1. Rupture or perforation of the gastrointestinal or biliary tracts.
2. Direct extension through the inflamed wall of the gastrointestinal tract or uterus.
3. Hematogenous in certain specific infectious diseases.

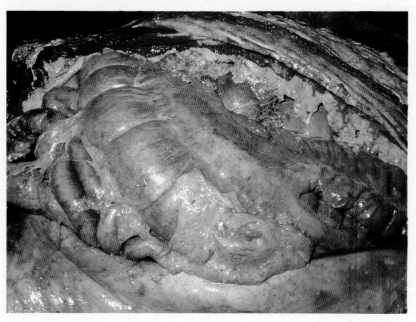

Plate 512   Equine Peritonitis

A ruptured viscus is the cause of fibrinous, gangrenous peritonitis.

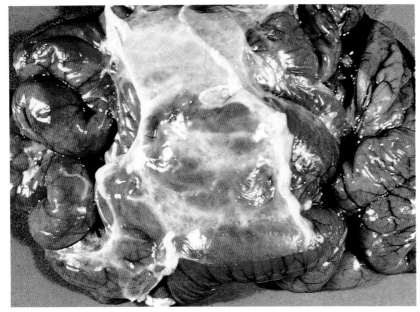

Plate 513   Glasser's Disease

Hematogenous dissemination of Haemophilus parasuis resulted in serofibrinous peritonitis in this weaner pig. Mycoplasma hyorhinis causes a similar peritonitis.

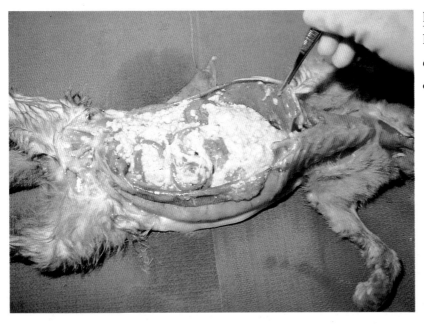

Plate 514   Feline Pasteurellosis

Patches of cream-colored, fibrinopurulent exudate cover the intestinal tract of a cat.

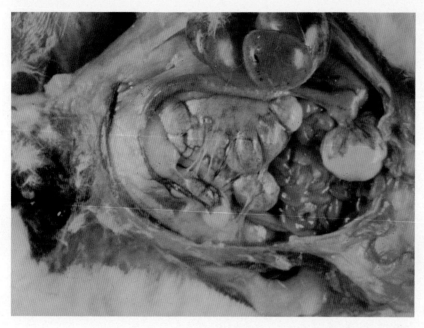

Plate 515 Rabbit Pasteurellosis

Large purulent nodules have disseminated within the abdominal cavity of an adult rabbit.

Feline Infectious Peritonitis (FIP)

FIP is a well described disease entity of domestic and wild Felidae. It is caused by a coronavirus. Although many cats are infected with the virus, relatively few cats develop the fatal form of the disease. "Wet" (effusive) and "dry" (non-effusive) are terms to describe the fatal forms of FIP infection. The disease is largely immune-mediated.

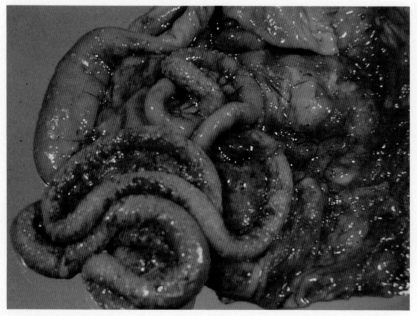

Plate 516 FIP

Grossly, a greyish-white granular exudate covers all serosal surfaces, and is especially thick over liver and spleen. In protracted cases, organization of the fibrinous exudate can result in severe distortion of abdominal viscera by fibrosis.

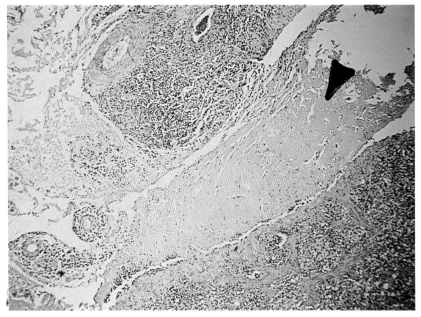

Plates 517,518   FIP

A pyogranuloma is the main histologic lesion in FIP. Neutrophils, lymphocytes and plasma cells have a tendency to accumulate around serosal vessels. Layers of fibrin (arrow) of varying thickness cover the surface of affected organs. The inflammatory process may extend below the serosa into the parenchyma of any of the affected organs. Vasculitis and perivasculitis are the results of antigen-antibody immune complex formations. H&E stain.

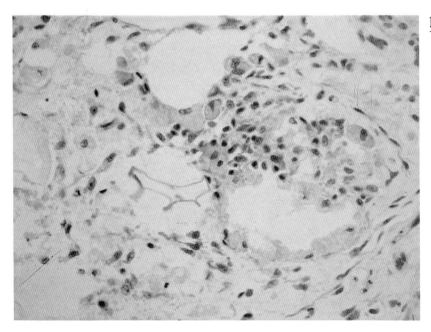

Plate 518   FIP

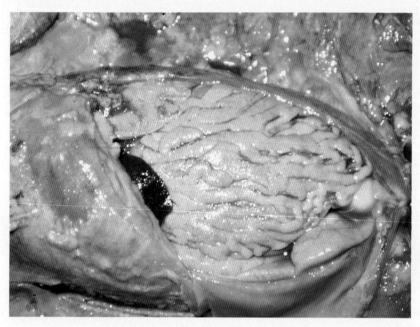

Plate 519   Nutritional Steatitis
Yellow fat disease (steatitis) in the cat is caused by hypovitaminosis E. The affected cats typically have been on fish diets only for some extended period of time. Pain and lumpiness of the subcutaneous tissue are clinical observations. The subcutaneous and abdominal adipose tissues are markedly discolored by yellow or brown ceroid pigments which act as irritant foreign bodies inciting an inflammatory reaction.

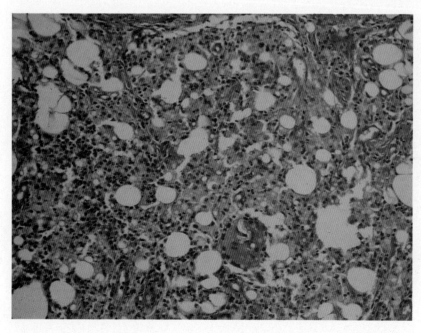

Plate 520   Nutritional Steatitis
Microscopically, fat necrosis, mineralization and a foreign-body inflammatory response are features of feline steatitis. H&E stain.

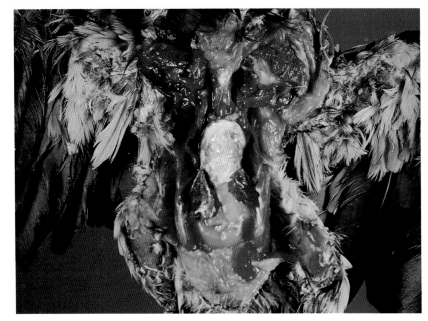

Plate 521   Mycotic Coelomitis

In birds, _Aspergillus_ sp. frequently are the cause of a disseminated, plaque-like, chalky exudate covering the serosal surfaces. The infection has to be differentiated from visceral gout.

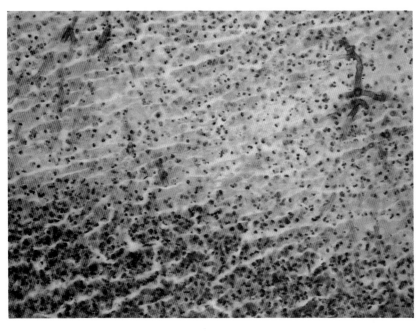

Plates 522,523   Mycotic Coelomitis

Ghost-like mycotic hyphae are visible within a coagulative exudate. H&E stain.

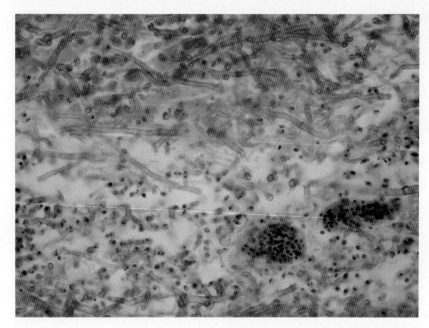

Plate 523   Mycotic Coelomitis

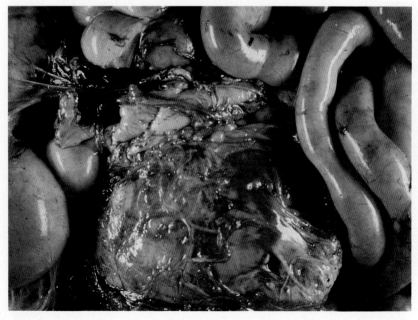

Plates 524,525   Bastard Strangles

Typically, strangles is an upper respiratory disease of horses caused by Streptococcus equi. Aberrant abscesses occasionally form in mesenteric lymph nodes. The lymph nodes may become quite large during this process and may cause fibrinous adhesions of adjacent viscera.

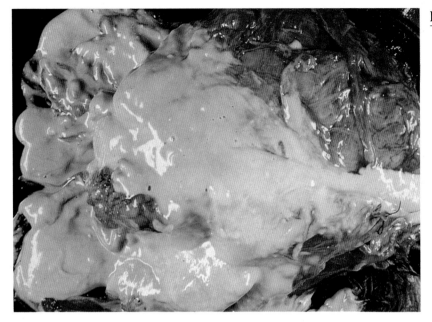

Plate 525   Bastard Strangles

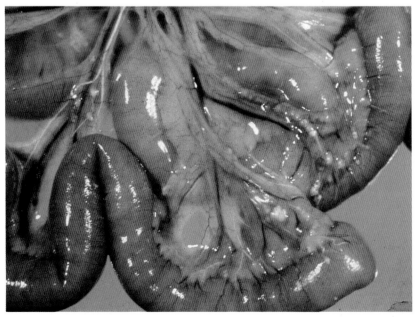

Plate 526   Lipogranulomatous Lymphangitis

A focal, necrotizing, granulomatous lymphangitis may accompany mesenteric lymphangiectasia in the dog.

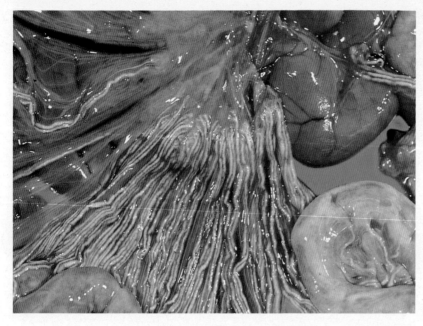

Plate 527 R. Equi Lymphangitis

A necrotizing polylymphangitis has occurred in a foal infected with R. equi.

III. Parasitic Peritonitis

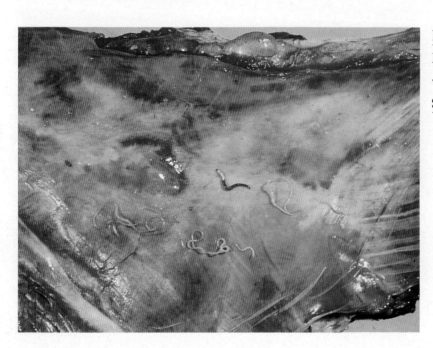

Plate 528 Equine Strongylosis

Larvae of Strongylus edentatus have invaded the parietal peritoneum of a horse.
Sertaria sp. are also present.

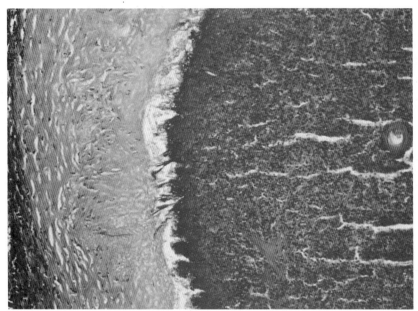

Plate 529   Equine Strongylosis

Microscopically, strongyle larvae have caused an eosinophilic abscess. H&E stain.

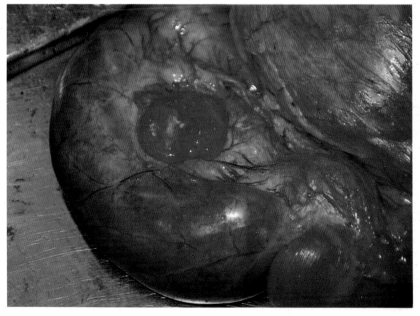

Plate 530   Ovine Cysticercosis

A fluid-filled cyst containing a single cestode (Cysticercus tenuicollis) larva is associated with the serosal surface of the abomasum of a sheep.

IV. Peritoneal Neoplasms

Mesotheliomas are primary neoplasm of the peritoneum arising from serosal cells. Most are seen in cattle and dogs, and most if not all are malignant. These tumors spread rapidly over the peritoneal surfaces giving rise to numerous small, variously shaped growths which grossly resemble tuberculous peritonitis ("Pearly Disease").

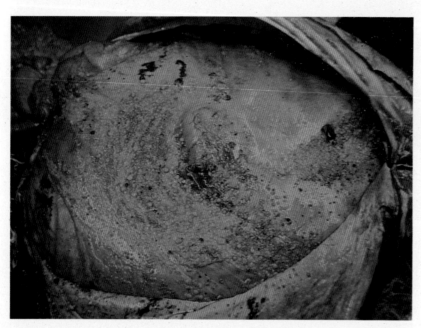

Plate 531 Mesothelioma

Malignant mesothelioma spreading over the visceral and parietal serosa in a calf. Ascites may develop, but unlike chronic granulomatous peritonitis, there are no adhesions. Calves may be born with this tumor.

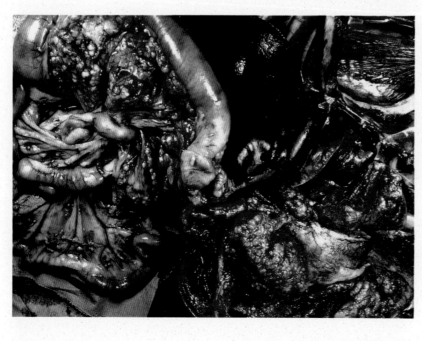

Plate 532 Mesothelioma

A granular, nodular growth has seeded the mesentery in a dog.

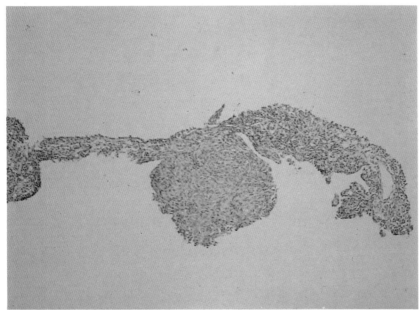

Plates 533,534 Mesothelioma

The tumor is composed of compact sheets of cuboidal, polygonal cells that form papillary projections and rest on a thin fibrous stroma. Mesothelioma is a misnomer in that this tumor has a malignant biological behavior. H&E stain.

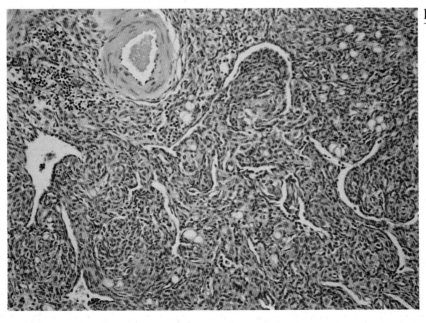

Plate 534 Mesothelioma

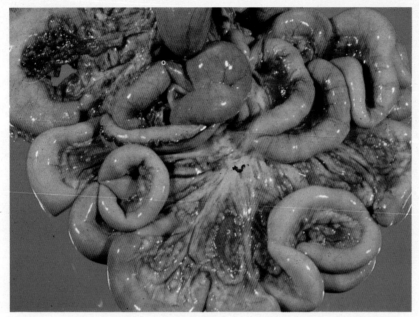

Plate 535 Secondary Peritoneal Tumors

Certain carcinomas tend to seed secondarily via implantation or lymphatic spread throughout the abdominal cavity. Some of these tumor cases may resemble chronic peritonitis as seen in this dog with prostatic carcinoma metastases.

Literature

1 . M.L. Harbison, J.J. Godleski: Malignant Mesothelioma in Urban Dogs. Vet. Path. 20:531, 1983.

2 . T. Hayashi, N. Goto, R. Takahashi, K. Fujiwana: Detection of Coronavirus-like Particles in a Spontaneous Case of Feline Infectious Peritonitis. Jap. J. Vet. Sci. 40:207, 1978.

3 . G.J. Schamber, C. Olson, L.E. Witt: Neoplasms in Calves. Vet. Path. 19:629, 1987.

4 . M. Stoeber: Mesotheliomas in Calves. Tieraerztl. Umsch. 45:743, 1990.

5 . H.J. vanKruiningen, G.E. Lees, D.W. Hayden, D.J. Meuten, W.A. Rogers: Lipogranulomatous Lymphangitis in Canine Intestinal Lymphangiectasia. Vet. Path. 21:377, 1984.

(Numbers refer to Plates and captions)

G

H

N

O

P

T

:   :